Find Your Happy

Find Your Happy

**A depressive's step by step guide for
long lasting joy and happiness**

A. Luetchford

ISBN-13: 9781530840052
ISBN-10: 1530840058
Library of Congress Control Number: 2016909677
CreateSpace Independent Publishing Platform
North Charleston, South Carolina

For James, who gave me my reason to live.

CONTENTS

HOW TO USE THIS BOOK

I have written this book in an attempt to bridge anecdotal stories with robust research into the effectiveness of certain activities, techniques, and strategies (interventions) for reducing the symptoms of depression.

Find Your Happy is designed for everyone. Whether you are severely depressed, feel a bit blue, or feel absolutely fine and dandy but want to practise self-care, this book is for you. We all want good mental health.

I want to play my part in reducing the stigma around mental illness, so have used my own story as a vehicle for this step-by-step guide. I realised that if I didn't share my experiences, I would feel complicit in silencing the conversation around mental health.

I've tried to ensure that this book is practical and based on evidence. I've also resisted the temptation to ruminate and have instead tried to put as many funny anecdotes in as possible—I do have a dark sense of humour. I want to show that I am human, that I don't always get things right, and that that is OK. No one is perfect. In fact, we are all perfectly *imperfect*.

There are certain steps that should be taken first (such as getting professional support as appropriate, and focusing on the fundamentals such as eating healthily, sleeping well, and exercising regularly) so that the interventions discussed in this book can work more effectively. But ultimately it's up to you to decide what works best. If you prefer to dip in and out of chapters, that's fine. If you prefer to read this cover to cover, that's also fine. This is your book.

Evidence-Based Interventions

The following organisations provide the most robust evidence on the effects of certain interventions for depression and their findings have been prioritised.

- Cochrane[1] is a global network of patients, researchers, professionals, and carers. Cochrane undertakes extremely high-quality meta-analyses of medical research to summarise the evidence base for interventions.

  The Cochrane Common Mental Health Disorders Group helpfully lists the interventions that have been analysed, along with summaries of the findings.[2]

---

1 "Cochrane," http://www.cochrane.org/. Accessed 27.06.2016.
2 "Cochrane: Common Mental Disorders," http://cmd.cochrane.org/our-work-0. Accessed 27.06.2016.

- The National Institute for Health and Care Excellence (NICE)[3] produces evidence-based guidance for health practitioners to improve health and social care.
- The Royal College of Psychiatrists is responsible for "education and training, and setting and raising standards in psychiatry."[4] Its website contains helpful information and advice.

While this book has been designed with any reader in mind (depressed or not), I have prioritised evidence about depression as it is the most relevant for the difficulties I describe. I have also prioritised evidence exploring the effects of interventions on adults rather than on adolescents, children, or the elderly. Again, this is because it is (a) most relevant for this book and (b) it is hard enough to find robust evidence for adults in general, let alone others.

Where there is evidence for a particular intervention, I have listed it. If there is no evidence, I have still included that intervention if it forms part of my story. Most of the time, the interventions worked for me. But it is completely up to you as to which interventions you want to try and I recommend prioritising interventions which evidence shows to be beneficial.

---

3 "NICE: National Institute for Health and Care Excellence," https://www.nice.org.uk/. Accessed 27.06.2016.

4 "Royal College of Psychiatrists," http://www.rcpsych.ac.uk/. Accessed 27.06.2016.

PROLOGUE

It was an ordinary, sunny May bank holiday weekend. Away from my husband and surrounded by close friends, I was relaxing after a successful art exhibition, eating and drinking at the Vegfest festival in Bristol. It was a beautiful weekend by anyone's standards.

But I suddenly felt an overwhelming desire to kill myself. A dark and dangerous monster had appeared; it had taken control of my soul and was intent on killing me. Suicide was both inviting and tempting. Contrary to what most people say about suicide, to me, at that point in time, killing myself was the most positive thing I could do. A liberation from my mind that would result in endless nothingness. I couldn't imagine anything better. During that weekend, suicide played on my mind constantly, like a song on repeat that I couldn't shake from my head. I imagined the specific ways I could kill myself in detail, like a foodie considering her next meal. I didn't know why, but everything about it just felt right. Completely right. And the urge to act on it was strong.

I didn't know what had triggered this desire or why it had been triggered at this particular moment. All I knew was that the dark emotions and urges were back, stronger and more dangerous than ever—because I knew exactly what to do. I had experienced these urges before during former episodes of mental illness over the previous decade but had fortunately been free of them for a couple of years. Until now.

Like the good researcher I was, I'd done my homework when depressed four years ago. I'd found a document online that explicitly described (nearly) every method for a successful suicide. Killing yourself isn't as easy as you might think and the potential for it to go wrong is huge. But I wanted to die. I'm going to say that again. I wanted to die. I wanted death. I wanted nothing apart from endless nothingness, endless peace. People freak out sometimes when you say you want to kill yourself. In fact, even just hearing the words "suicide" or "death" can be enough to make people run a mile in the opposite direction. It's not socially appropriate to talk of such things, not polite dinner party chitchat. I'd always found it odd that my therapists were the ones who truly knew me the best. I could say anything to them, and they wouldn't leave or tell me off for saying such things. I could talk about death in detail, and they would let me talk undisturbed. Thinking about death was such a large part of my life that it had been my secret plan B for over ten years.

But my ever-present plan B had now been bumped up to plan A. I didn't want to fail and give myself organ failure or go into a vegetative state. I wanted my death to be as easy, successful, and pain-free as possible. And I didn't want to be stopped.

Because I'd had these feelings before, the rational part of my mind (what was left of it) knew these thoughts weren't what others would consider "normal." Rather than secretly planning ways to act on them as I had in the past, my rational mind understood these feelings for what they were: symptoms of my depression, stress, and anxiety. They were telling me that I needed professional help, and fast. But I wasn't at home to get that help.

I was staying with friends, trying to have my fun weekend. I was away from home, and most importantly, away from my husband. I hadn't yet told him about my previous suicide attempts, but I knew I needed his help. And fast.

I was safe with my friends. I knew that my death would be traumatic enough without them having to find me or clean up the mess. In my unbalanced and irrational state, I didn't want to put them out by killing myself when I was with them. Instead, I wanted to kill myself while I was at home, undisturbed. Considerate, that.

I'd planned a day for my suicide a few times before. I'd even tried it a couple of times before. It's odd, trying to find time to kill yourself. My diary was always packed, and finding a slot was a challenge. I tried to distract myself with retail therapy but realised after I'd got into town that it was pointless buying clothes. The money would be more helpful to my family in my bank. It's amazing what goes through your mind when you're not well.

So instead, I phoned my husband and began to speak honestly and openly. There were a lot of tears—distressed, concerned tears. I desperately wanted to be with him. I knew I'd be safe with him. But I was a hundred miles away.

Getting Help

If you or anyone you know has a mental-health concern, visit a health professional such as your GP.

If you or anyone you know feels suicidal, call 999 or visit Accident & Emergency, where you can talk to professionals who will be able to help.

When I did get home, I knew I had to get help—fast. I could go to A&E, but what I really needed was time off work and medication. A lot of medication. And my GP was best placed for prescribing that.

But our GP had a new booking system, meaning that in order to see someone that day, I had to wait in line with other people at 7:40 a.m., ready for the doors to open at 8:00 a.m. It's strange, queuing up with Joe Bloggs when you're trying to keep yourself alive yet simultaneously planning how you're going to die. I was glad that the GP surgery wasn't by a busy street because I had a strong urge to walk out in front of any vehicle going fast enough. I also was strongly tempted to jump in front of a train. Guess I wasn't going to be taking the London Underground anytime soon then.

I was one of the lucky ones who got a telephone appointment. It helped that I told the receptionist I was actively suicidal. I hate GP receptions. There is rarely privacy to communicate about sensitive subjects. The only upside to the experience was that the receptionist was nicer after I'd said that. I find it amusing telling people when I feel suicidal. It's odd watching them react in such an uncomfortable way when my suicidal thoughts have been such a normal part of my everyday life for so many years. My plan B is like any good friend—the thought of suicide has stuck by me through thick and thin.

But instead of giving in to my plan B, I went home and called in sick because of my mental health for the first time in my professional career. And waited.

Eventually, the GP called. She was patient, empathic, understanding and prescribed new medication. I'd already tried a handful of different medications over the years with varying side effects. Fluoxetine (Prozac) had made me actively suicidal which wasn't ideal for someone severely depressed. Mirtazapine had increased my appetite, leading me to put on a stone within six weeks, plus it turned me into a sleeping zombie who was only awake four hours a day. Citalopram had generally been good, but after I tried it for a second time, it had lost its effectiveness.

So I ended up on sertraline. Unusually, its side effects were quite nice. Initially experiencing insomnia (very useful in terms of productivity), I then experienced symptoms similar to hypomania (again, very enjoyable), plus I felt drunk for a week (awesome). Oh, and I lost a stone in weight. Pills that made me happier, gave me energy, and helped me to lose weight—what more could I want?

I knew in my heart, body, and mind that I needed time off work to get better. During previous suicidal episodes, I'd carried on working, but the urges hadn't been as strong or as dark then. After hearing my GP suggest two to three weeks, I decided to take the least amount of time. After all, I'd be back at work soon, wouldn't I?

RECOVER

CANCEL LIFE

was brilliant at getting things done. I was Miss Proactive, Miss Organised, and Miss Perfectionist all rolled into one—a deadly combination. My weekly diary was a beautiful sight: every single errand and task to do was noted down in glorious detail and was duly ticked off as each mission was accomplished. Accomplishing tasks gave me a sense of purpose; I'd achieved something and felt I was worth something. And why leave something for tomorrow when it could be done today? After all, no one else would do it for me.

Not only did these tasks have to be done, they had to be done to the unreasonably high standard that I had set for myself. Anything less, and I was disappointed in myself. I hadn't performed as I should have and had done something substandard. I was worse than average.

I'd always been "busy," primarily because I believed being busy had helpfully sped up my childhood. Stuck in an English boarding school while my parents were living in America, I hated term time. In fact, I hated term time so much that aged just eleven, half my hair fell out due to stress. What child should experience that? Despite my daily teary and heartfelt telephone calls to my parents to let me live with them, I was left in England. And they remained in America.

The only saving grace was that I was allowed home during the summer holidays. After my first idyllic and beautiful American summer holiday and facing an overnight flight back to London's Heathrow, I was overcome with a sense of waste. I'd wasted my summer. I had nothing to show for all the time I'd spent there, and I couldn't differentiate one day from another in my memory. I thought this was a Very Bad Thing. I had lost something I could never recover. I wouldn't realise for decades that my summer had been perfect just the way it was. I had spent time with my family, read numerous books, and swum in our local pool during those hot afternoons. As an adult looking back, I couldn't have planned a better or more restful summer holiday.

But aged eleven, I felt ashamed. Believing I'd wasted those precious two months, I promised myself that I would accomplish something every single day. I would make every day of my life "count." Plus being busy would help time go faster, meaning I'd escape school faster. Win-win. And so my years on the treadmill started.

■ ■ ■

Fast-forward twenty years. Despite my husband's best attempts at trying to help me relax and reduce my social commitments, I was still an active "doer." No task was too small for this woman! I'd learnt how to fix (some parts of) my car, redecorated our flat, planned our wedding, and was kick-starting my art career around a full-time and stressful day job. Oh, and my husband had been diagnosed as disabled, meaning that I now had caring responsibilities and had to help him navigate the world of limited welfare benefits.

Friends knew that in order to see me, they had to schedule time three weeks in advance, and even then there was no guarantee that I would be free. Colleagues had to book time in my (jam-packed) diary if they wanted a chat. I didn't waste a single minute and employed numerous business strategies and techniques to maximise my efficiency. I was the queen of multitasking. Lunch breaks were perfect for exercising or personal admin tasks. Evenings were filled with painting and developing my art business. Weekends were often social affairs, although I remembered little afterwards. I accounted for every second and made each and every one as efficient as possible. I had action plans, to-do lists, and diary entries seeping into every area of my life.

I was on a treadmill, living the supposed "dream." I had my own flat, a wonderful husband, and a demanding but (mostly) rewarding day job. What else did a woman need? Surely I had everything I was told I needed by society and its invasive marketing. While I couldn't afford the boozy and entertainment-driven lifestyle other fellow London professionals could, I made up for it by being "busy" every single minute. I was productive. I was worthy. Yet I wasn't happy.

I was stressed. At work, feeling undervalued and over-worked, I rarely even found time to go to the loo. Emails from my manager induced panic and terror. The sight of a new email in my inbox was enough to send my stress lev-els sky-high with the anticipation of what that email might contain. Too many times an email contained a data "emer-gency" that needed sorting out yesterday. I would hyper-ventilate and try not to pass out at my desk by resting my head on my arm. I would flee to the loo to cry quietly. (The disabled loo is always best for this, silent and undis-turbed.) I wept as I cycled to work, scaring the pigeons. I sometimes wept at the thought of work. But I was liv-ing the "dream," right? Everyone else had a stressful job, didn't they? Wasn't it a badge of honour to always be busy, work long hours, and be constantly stressed? Maybe I just couldn't cope. Maybe I was weak. Maybe it was my fault I was so unhappy. Maybe I was to blame.

I was miserable. I always concentrated on the next activity at hand and rarely, if ever, mindfully enjoyed or appreciated the present moment. I'm ashamed to admit that when meeting my nearest and dearest friends, I spent too much of my time thinking and worrying about what I was meant to do next. Telephone calls to family fell by the wayside. I didn't have any time to process what I was doing, collect my thoughts, or gain perspective about life as a whole. The treadmill kept turning and I didn't know how to get off.

■ ■ ■

Being signed off work sick due to mental illness was the tangible sign I needed to acknowledge there was (a) something seriously wrong and (b) a need to make radical changes. Sickness had given me the "permission" I sought to cancel plans and prioritise my health. But my mistake had been waiting until I had become very sick. Until then, I hadn't thought I deserved to prioritise myself above others. I was a "nice" person, a people pleaser who always put others' needs before mine. And my own needs had fallen by the wayside.

But things had to change. It's odd, being off sick from work because of mental illness. What should you do all day? Lying in bed wasn't really an option and would not have been conducive to a positive recovery either. Instead, together with my husband, I realised I had to:

a. Do Only What's Pleasurable or Necessary

In Essentialism, *Greg McKeown explains that it is critical to both limit the number of things you do, and to have the space and time to do them well and enjoy them. He describes thorough and practical ways of practising "essentialism,"[5] including techniques for saying no.*

Paul Gilbert uses research and evidence from a broad range of disciplines to explain the importance of being

5 Greg McKeown, *Essentialism: The Disciplined Pursuit of Less* (United Kingdom: Virgin Books, 2014).

self-compassionate in The Compassionate Mind.[6] *The second half of the book describes helpful techniques for practising self-compassion.*

These feats were both easier and harder than I expected. It's wonderfully simple to cancel all plans—I just texted or emailed people to explain that I wasn't well. The responses I got were wonderfully understanding and supportive. My family and friends respected my honesty. They wanted me to be happy and healthy and therefore supported my steps towards being so.

Yet doing only things that I enjoyed or had to do was much harder than I had anticipated. First of all, because I had been prioritising others' needs above my own, I struggled to actually know what I enjoyed for myself. How did I spend my days when I had free time? I came to realise that my own happiness was very linked to a sense of purpose rather than pleasure[7]—contributing to the sense that I was on a constant and never-slowing treadmill. I had spent my free time running errands in order to feel purposeful, but I had totally neglected the activities I enjoyed just because they made me *happy*. In fact, I had ignored them so much that I didn't know what they actually were. I had to go back to basics and learn what made me happy.

6 Paul Gilbert, *The Compassionate Mind: Compassion Focused Therapy* (United Kingdom: Constable, 2009).
7 Paul Dolan, *Happiness by Design: Change What You Do, Not How You Think* (United Kingdom: Penguin, 2014).

The depression didn't make it easy. I frequently struggled to feel *anything*. I often felt I *should* be happy during certain occasions, but the reality was that I rarely did. Instead, I felt numb at best and desperately wretched at worst. Even if I appeared happy on the surface, it was a (probably not very convincing) mask.

My first task—yes, another task—was to find out what I actually enjoyed. I started writing a daily journal, where I listed:

i)   Things I had enjoyed that day
ii)   Things I had not enjoyed that day
iii) Areas I wanted to focus on the following day
iv)   Things I was grateful for

The act of writing lists for these four categories was a revelation. Being honest with myself, I realised that I often enjoyed the simple things in life: curling up with a cup of tea and a magazine, cuddling the cat, or watching a good film with my husband. I didn't enjoy activities that many others did: drinking in bars, clubbing, or socialising in large groups. Noise and crowds were unsettling and often frightening, plus I'd given up alcohol, which made many environments duller than before.

But more interesting was my realisation about the *people* I felt happy to be around—and didn't. While I wasn't able to socialise for a month (it took me that long to look someone in the eye), when I was healthier, I became fascinated with how socialising made me feel. Some people made me feel warm and fuzzy inside; others drained me and made me more stressed and sad. So I proactively limited time with the latter and sought out time with the former. Brutal but necessary.

I also hid all Facebook posts from people who didn't make me feel happier. Neutral Facebook posts weren't enough; I could read only positive posts.

Project Happy had begun.

Each day my husband and I identified one single activity we could do that I would enjoy. My energy levels weren't high, and I was uncomfortable being around other people, so our excursions had to be short and full of pleasure. I was adjusting to the side effects of my new medication, which made me feel drunk when out and about, which was really rather nice!

Many of our activities revolved around cake. While I felt sick and dizzy, the only food that appealed to me was cake. As I was not renowned for having a hugely sweet tooth previously, this was a change for me. Perhaps it was the lack of sugar after giving up alcohol, but ever since I'd become ill, I'd craved cake. Victoria sponge, lemon drizzle, carrot cake, cheesecake, vegan cake, non-vegan cake…I loved cake. Each excursion was better with a planned tea-and-cake stop. Delicious.

Another activity I enjoyed was seeing art exhibitions. I wasn't required to walk long distances (my energy levels being problematic), I didn't have to engage with other people, and I'd always loved being surrounded by and creating art. We saw exhibition after exhibition after exhibition.

And when things became too much, when I had been in Central London for too long, I would run away back to our flat and paint. No matter how difficult the excursion had been, no matter how panicked, stressed, or anxious I'd become, painting soothed me and was a balm to my troubled soul. It didn't matter what I painted, just that I painted. And painted. And painted some more.

FOCUS ON THE FUNDAMENTALS

b. Sleep

The National Institute for Health and Care Excellence (NICE) recommends that people with depression practise positive sleep hygiene. This includes:

- *"establishing regular sleep and wake times*
- *avoiding excess eating, smoking, or drinking alcohol before sleep*
- *creating a proper environment for sleep*
- *taking regular physical exercise."* [8]

The Royal College of Psychiatrists recommends finding other ways of relaxing if sleep itself is too difficult.[9]

---

8 NICE, "Depression in Adults: Recognition and Management," last modified 2016, https://www.nice.org.uk/guidance/cg90/chapter/1-Guidance#step-1-recognition-assessment-and-initial-management.

9 Royal College of Psychiatrists, "Depression" (2016), http://www.rcpsych.ac.uk/healthadvice/problemsdisorders/depression.aspx.

I'd long ago known that I needed to focus on the fundamentals, which were sleeping, eating well, and exercising. This knowledge was reinforced by nearly every professional I'd seen during depressive episodes—and I'd seen many. Psychologists, psychiatrists, GPs, psycho- and CBT therapists, counsellors, A&E staff, mental-health nurses, crisis teams—I'd seen them all.

But in my downward spiral, caring for myself was the last thing on my mind. Instead, I wanted to punish myself. I wanted to inflict the pain on myself that I believed I deserved. But while I might not have appreciated it at the time, focusing on the fundamentals was key. It might not solve every single problem, but it's a damn good foundation on which to build positive mental health.

Ironically, the side effects of my medication made it harder for me to look after myself. Initially I suffered insomnia. My mind raced, keeping me up for hours throughout the night. I felt hyped up, wired, and unable to concentrate during the day. My shoulders were rigid and sore with stress, and my jaw was clenched tight. When I did finally manage to sleep, I woke up my husband as I loudly ground my teeth. Not ideal for either of us.

But then the insomnia and adrenaline wore off, and I started to sleep. And sleep some more. I realised that as with a physical illness, my body needed to rest and recover, and sleeping was a wonderful way to temporarily escape my mind and all of its negativity. Plus, sleeping made me more able to cope with the following day. I'd always struggled when I was tired, feeling more emotional and sensitive and less resilient. Small setbacks felt like mountains to overcome, and the slightest negative remark delivered a sharp and hefty blow to my fragile sense of self. But after a good night's sleep, I found I was usually emotionally stronger and retained perspective more easily. I was far more likely to be able to respond positively to any situation.

c. Eat Healthily (and Avoid Alcohol)

The Royal College of Psychiatrists recommends eating healthily as "Depression can make you lose weight and run short of vitamins which will only make you feel worse. Fresh fruit and vegetables are particularly helpful." It also notes that "Alcohol actually makes depression worse. It may make you feel better for a short while, but it doesn't last. Drinking can stop you dealing with important problems and from getting the right help. It's also bad for your physical health."[10]

The National Health Service (NHS) advises patients with stress, anxiety, or depression to try to eat a healthy diet and not consume too much alcohol.[11]

---

10 Royal College of Psychiatrists, "Depression," *Health Advice, Problems & Disorders* (June 2015), http://www.rcpsych.ac.uk/healthadvice/problemsdisorders/depression.aspx. Accessed 27.06.2016.

11 National Health Service (NHS), "Tips for coping with depression," last reviewed January 2016, http://www.nhs.uk/conditions/stress-anxiety-depression/pages/dealing-with-depression.aspx.

I also changed my diet. Apart from the (daily) cake, I tried to eat healthily to fuel my body with the most nutritious and beneficial food I could. No ready meals or takeaways for me—I wanted vitamins, minerals, and a balanced diet of goodness to give my body and mind the best chance possible of recovering. I experimented with different types of food and tried to be vegan where possible[12]—with, of course, the exception of cake.

And buffets. I must also admit here that I developed an unhealthy obsession with all-you-can-eat buffets. But I wasn't interested in one single cuisine; I wanted a range: Chinese, Indian, American, Italian, French, English—you name it, I wanted it. After an embarrassingly large amount of research, I was disillusioned with the options London had to offer, and so cast my net wider.

I grew up in Bath, and many of my friends and family members now live in the Bath/Bristol area. I'd heard about Za Za Bazaar, an all-you-can-eat, globally inspired buffet restaurant in the centre of Bristol. At £8.99 for a weekday lunch, it was astoundingly good value. So we went. It turns out that a National Express coach ticket plus the £8.99 for lunch are cheaper than many London-based food options, and we had the added bonus that my sister-in-law could join us as well. We had the time, so feeling rather like day-tripping pensioners and armed with reading material, we boarded the bus to Bristol.

---

12 For environmental reasons rather than specific health reasons.

It was wonderful. I ate an extraordinary amount. Guests are only allowed an hour and forty-five minutes per sitting, so the clock was ticking. Unfortunately for my husband and sister-in-law, my focus was on eating, and therefore my already limited (due to the medication) conversation skills were even more limited during the lunch. Five plates of cheesecake later, I was finished. I was not quite the same size or shape as I was before I entered, as my husband kindly pointed out, but I was very happy. Relieved too that we'd had the foresight to plan an hour before we boarded our coach back to London so that we could lie down in the park until we felt slightly less sick. Slightly. It was a great day.

After our visit to Za Za Bazaar, I experimented with veganism. My attempts at vegan cooking provided both my husband and me with unexpected yet surprisingly regular periods of hilarity. I made brownies out of sweet potatoes and black beans, scones so hard they were inedible, and banana bread so chewy it was more similar to chewing gum than bread. I learnt the hard way that (a) you have to have all the right ingredients for vegan baking and (b) you have to put them all in the mixing bowl. Otherwise it just doesn't work. In fact, I had so many disasters that when speaking to my husband about this book, he helpfully suggested including a list of dishes that had gone well rather than those that hadn't, as the former would be shorter. Sod.

I also made the decision to stop drinking alcohol, both because it could interfere with my medication and because alcohol is a depressant—not conducive to a fast or productive recovery from a major depressive episode. I had been drinking socially before I'd become ill, but drinking increased the chances that I'd argue with my husband. I also found I would be riddled with angst the following day, reliving conversations (when I could remember them) and fearing that I'd offended someone. If I wasn't reassured that I'd acted in an acceptable way, I would assume I'd been a horrible person to my nearest and dearest and feel terrible about myself. I looked for as many ways to beat myself up as I could.

Because of these reasons and because I was the sole earner in the household, needing to return to work as soon as I possibly could for financial reasons, I decided to go completely cold turkey and embrace sobriety.

Twelve months later, I now don't want to drink alcohol at all. After not drinking for the two months I was signed off work, I just haven't been tempted to start again. I appreciate the more balanced moods, the lack of anxiety, and the health benefits. I sleep like a baby every single night without the early morning hangovers or tossing and turning in a drunken, light sleep. And if I do fancy the taste of a glass of wine or beer, then there is a growing market of nonalcoholic beer and wine that actually taste like beer and wine.[13] Half the price, fewer than half the calories, and I don't have to worry about acting foolishly—what's not to love?

---

13 The best nonalcoholic beer I've found is San Miguel's 0.0%, and the best nonalcoholic wines I've found are Eisberg wines, particularly the Sauvignon Blanc and Merlot.

d. Exercise[14]

There is some research to show that exercise can be slightly beneficial for depression. The Cochrane Common Mental Disorders Group analysed the effects of exercise for depression. It found that exercise is "moderately more effective than no therapy for reducing symptoms of depression." However, when only including high-quality studies, "the difference between exercise and no therapy is less conclusive."

A small number of studies reviewed by the group found that exercise is "no more effective than antidepressants" or "psychological therapies for reducing symptoms of depression."[15]

The third fundamental step was to exercise gently. Always the "doer," I'd exercised regularly since 2009, cycling, running, and lifting weights. But my mental illness meant it was incredibly difficult to attend gym classes. I didn't want to speak to anyone, and being around others made me feel physically uncomfortable and panicky. I was scared of seeing people I knew in case they wanted to interact with me. Pretending to be "normal" while out and about took all the energy I had and more. So instead I took the

---

14 NHS, "Exercise for Depression," last modified January 2016, http://www.nhs.uk/Conditions/stress-anxiety-depression/Pages/Exercise-for-depression.aspx.

15 Gary Cooney, et al., "Exercise for Depression," *Cochrane Database of Systematic Reviews 2013*, Issue 9, Art. No.: CD004366, doi: 10.1002/14651858.CD004366.pub6, http://onlinelibrary.wiley.com/doi/10.1002/14651858.CD004366.pub6/full.

time to rest up and go for gentle walks with my husband. Gradually, as I became more emotionally balanced and able to interact with others, I returned to the gym. And when I felt even better, I managed to return to the more sociable gym classes. Slowly but surely, I was starting to rebuild my life.

CREATE SPACE TO BREATHE

e. Meditate

Research from the 1950s into the benefits of meditation has yielded varied results. Previous research was limited by poor methodology, which has limited the conclusions drawn from the results.[16]

My mind was working at full speed. Used to multitasking and working at a frenetic pace, I was unused to relaxing and resting. Consumed with anxious and negative thoughts, I was constantly beating myself up and was my own harshest critic. I was unable to attend doctors' appointments alone because I wasn't rational. My (long-suffering) husband accompanied me to every therapy and medical appointment, liaised with my line manager, and ensured that my targets for returning to work were realistic. When

---

16 Maria. B. Ospina, et al., "Clinical Trials of Meditation Practices in Health Care: Characteristics and Quality," *J Altern Complement Med* 14, no. 10 (December 2008): 1199–213, doi:10.1089/acm.2008.0307. http://online. liebertpub.com/doi/abs/10.1089/acm.2008.0307?journalCode=acm.

I was too optimistic about when I could return to work, he rightly and firmly told me I needed more time to recover before I was well enough to work again.

I needed to find a way to calm down.

So I tried meditating. Full of good intentions, I downloaded not only the Calm[17] app but also Headspace.[18] Unfortunately, downloading these apps didn't mean I was automatically able to meditate; apparently I had to remain still for that to happen. And that wasn't easy at all in my hyper and fidgety state. Nor was I comfortable spending time with my own thoughts—they scared me with their negativity and power. So I decided to try something else.

f. Dance

There is very limited research into the benefits of 5Rhythms dance; in fact, there is currently only one research paper discussing a small-scale research project.[19]

The Cochrane Common Mental Disorders Group has investigated the effects of dance/movement therapy and notes that there is "no evidence for or against DMT as a treatment for depression. There is some evidence to

17 https://www.calm.com/.

18 https://www.headspace.com/.

19 Sarah Cook, Karen Ledger, and Nadine Scott, *Dancing for Living Report: Women's Experience of 5 Rhythms Dance and the Effects on Their Emotional Wellbeing* (Sheffield: UK Advocacy Network, 2003).

suggest DMT is more effective than standard care for adults, but this was not clinically significant."[20]

I decided to try dancing, specifically the meditative dance/movement practice 5Rhythms.[21] Introduced to it by a friend, I found it was a great way to respond to music in a free and soothing way—dancing in whichever manner the music inspired me, guided by a skilful facilitator. However, while I loved the principles of it, I struggled with a whole (two-and-a-half-hour) class. My energy levels depleted rapidly, and I was soon exhausted. Plus, being around so many people was just intimidating. Because I'd loved the feeling of dancing, just not for a whole class, I instead tried to dance to music at home.

My attempts at home were disastrous. Unable to find specific 5Rhythms music, I decided to use my own playlist. Slightly too enthusiastically, I promptly started prancing around to the most uplifting and gorgeous songs I could find as I dressed in the morning. But unfortunately I didn't realise my hair straighteners had become quite so hot, and I decided to give it a rest after I'd burnt my scalp. Multitasking just isn't all it's cracked up to be.

---

20 Bonnie Meekums, Vicky Karkou, and E. Andrea Nelson, "Is Dance Movement Therapy an Effective Treatment for Depression? A Review of the Evidence," *Cochrane Database of Systematic Reviews 2015, Issue 2*, Art. No.: CD009895, doi: 10.1002/14651858.CD009895.pub2 (February 2015). http://onlinelibrary.wiley.com/doi/10.1002/14651858.CD009895.pub2/abstract.

21 https://en.wikipedia.org/wiki/5Rhythms.

g. Practise Yoga

Recent research in Australia explored the benefits of seventeen natural therapies for depression. After analysing 67 reviews on a total of 111 randomised control trials, the authors concluded that there was weak evidence to show that yoga was beneficial for people with depression. However, there was a lack of studies and information, and where RCTs had been undertaken, they contained design and reporting issues.[22]

I decided to turn my attention to something slower and calmer: yoga. A close friend recommended it to me, and after hearing that she could now (a) do the splits and (b) was having better sex, I was intrigued. But I wasn't yet up to going to a yoga class, so instead took a more home-based approach and decided to try Yoga with Adriene[23] on YouTube.

It's worth pointing out that my only previous experience of yoga had been in India with a close friend, who I'll call H. While that sounds exotic and successful, it wasn't. Our one and only session was in McLeod Ganj, set high in the Himalayan mountain range and boasting stunning and inspirational views. The very kind yet

---

22 Chris Baggoley, *Review of the Australian Government Rebate on Natural Therapies for Private Health Insurance* (Australian Government—Department of Health, 2015), http://www.health.gov.au/internet/main/publishing.nsf/Content/0E9129B3574FCA53CA257BF0001ACD11/$File/Natural%20Therapies%20Overview%20Report%20Final%20with%20copyright%2011%20March.pdf.

23 https://www.youtube.com/user/yogawithadriene.

quickly dismayed yoga teacher explained he wasn't used to teaching Europeans and was fascinated by my lack of flexibility. H took a slightly different approach, preferring a horrified reaction to my (lack of) bodily contortions. In fact, the whole experience left such an imprint on my memory that I never tried yoga again.

Until now.

I bought a mat online and started practising yoga daily. Adriene was gentle, supportive, and kind, and slowly but surely I began to loosen up. She mixed deep and restorative breathing with healing and soothing stretches for the body. Over the days, weeks, and months, my body and mind started to work closer together but at a slower speed. I was able to breathe. And prioritising yoga reaffirmed to my (fragile) ego that I deserved to look after myself by nourishing my mind and body. I felt I was slowly healing.

h. Write

Expressive writing as a form of therapy started in the late 1980s, driven by James W. Pennebaker, who studied the effects of writing about past traumas.[24] Pennebaker found that those who had written continuously for fifteen minutes a day for four days in a row about a past trauma vis-

---

24 J. W. Pennebaker and S. K. Beall, "Confronting a Traumatic Event: Toward an Understanding of Inhibition and Disease," *Journal of Abnormal Psychology* 95, no. 3 (August 1986): 274–81.

ited their doctor less in the following months than those who had written about other subjects.

Although I was on my path to recovery, the critical voices in my head just wouldn't stop. While they were quieter and less frequent, they still persisted with negative and unkind thoughts and wore me down. So I built on the daily mental-health exercises I'd been doing in my journal and alternated them with entries of 750 words.[25] Originally from her book *The Artist's Way*,[26] Julia Cameron's concept of writing 750 words every morning (her morning pages) has grown in popularity throughout the world as its own concept.

The concept is simple. Every morning, write 750 words, or three pages, in your journal. While Julia Cameron recommends writing by hand, I find typing faster and therefore it is easier for my subconscious to speak. The thought of writing 750 words every day can be daunting, but it doesn't matter what you write about – only that you write. You might write "blah" 750 times. That's OK.

I haven't always been a writer and wouldn't even consider myself to be one now (despite what this book might

---

25 The 750 Words website (http://750words.com) offers an online tool to make the journaling process easier. Julia suggests writing three pages by hand every day, whereas 750 Words acknowledges that some people may find typing easier and so offers a space to write 750 words (equivalent to three pages of longhand). The website analyses the content you write and feeds back information, such as the moods you've expressed. Also offering motivational badges, it's the go-to place for anyone interested in this idea.
26 Julia Cameron, *The Artist's Way: A Course in Discovering and Recovering Your Creative Self* (UK: Souvenir Press Ltd., 1994).

indicate), so I admit I was sceptical at first. Before I started writing my morning pages, I preferred to draw or to chat with someone. But having given this a go, I've found that writing has a special power that I haven't found elsewhere. When I first start writing, my conscious mind will chatter away very happily. In fact, my dad once described my writing as verbal diarrhoea on a page. Charming. Writing helps me think things through, ponder quandaries, and often find solutions to problems.

But when my conscious voice quietens, something magical happens: my subconscious voice starts to talk. Strange anxieties surface that had previously been submerged. Issues float up that I had no idea were even bothering me. My mind is free to go in any which way it wants through the words I write.

If I am anxious about something, the journal is also a good space to articulate the anxiety and attempt to rationalise it. If it's a justified anxiety, then I might write down potential solutions and how they make me feel. If it's an unjustified anxiety, I can explain to myself why it doesn't count.

Journaling is a quick way to reflect on the day and identify the activities that spark happiness—or don't. Sometimes the results are expected; other times they surprise me. What I think makes me happy doesn't always, and sometimes I can appreciate the simplest of things. Nothing can beat curling up on the sofa with a blanket, cat, magazine, and cup of tea! Being honest about what I enjoy means I can do more of what I love and eliminate the things I don't. And my self-esteem and confidence have increased as I've started thinking and acting in a more authentic way, true to myself.

After journaling, my mind is clear and empty. The thoughts and feelings are transferred out of my mind and safely onto paper. The negative voice has stopped talking, and I have energy and space to take on the day. If I haven't been able to write for a day or two, I noticeably miss it and feel my mind filling with weird and wonderful information that hasn't been processed or filed away.

Sometimes I don't have time to write 750 words, and so I take another approach. As discussed before (and expanded slightly here), I do what I call my mental-health exercises in a journal by my bed. In it I list:

i)   Things that made me happy that day and how they made me feel
ii) Things that didn't make me happy that day and how they made me feel
iii) Areas that I want to focus on for the next day (such as pacing myself or focusing on one task at once)
iv) Things I feel proud of doing
v)   Things I'm grateful for

I return to my writing on a regular basis not because I feel I "should" or have to but because I want to. And am more balanced as a result.

PRIORITISE

i. Simplify Your Life

As mentioned before, McKeown's Essentialism *provides a helpful guide for prioritising and simplifying.*[27]

I was a conscientious, motivated perfectionist—a combination perfect for burnout.

I always aimed to complete every one of my tasks to a perfect standard. I didn't need to be motivated by others; my own internal standards were exceptionally and impossibly high. My grampa told me that if something was worth doing, it was worth doing well, so I aimed to do everything well. Every little task my manager suggested I do, I did. I wanted to outperform her expectations and my work objectives, always aiming to achieve that ever-elusive top performance rating.

Not only was I pressuring myself, but I felt pressured by the organisation too. There was always a huge amount of work that had to be done immediately. I didn't just

---

27 http://gregmckeown.com/.

work at a normal pace; I raced to my next activity. The only certainty was change, and if I didn't keep up, I could leave.

My job as a social researcher had also shifted, catapulting me further and further away from my comfort zone. My introverted mind loved data analysis, occasional teamwork, and the chance to be creative. But I was doing more and more public speaking, training, and designing software, none of which excited or motivated me. In fact, these activities made me feel like a failure. I didn't have enough background knowledge at that point to be confident in my abilities (although even if I had, my self-doubt was so strong that I would still have doubted myself). I felt as though I was underperforming at every step. As Einstein once said, everybody is a genius, but if you judge a fish on its ability to climb a tree, it will live its whole life believing that it is stupid. Well, I was the fish, and these new activities were my tree. In fact, they were more than just a tree; they were the biggest frigging trees in the forest.

Speaking up wasn't an option. My crippled self-esteem told me I wasn't enough secure enough in my job to challenge the workload or pace of change. I had been warned in the interview that the workload was high, so the rare times I initially had spoken up, I was told that I knew what I had let myself in for. As I did more and more tasks out of my comfort zone, my self-esteem dropped even further, I doubted my abilities more, and I enjoyed work less. It was a negative and self-perpetuating cycle.

I couldn't prioritise my tasks, as everything had to be done. Plus the stress had blinkered me; I had lost perspective and was completely unable to see the important from the unimportant. I was given data questions to answer within hours, requests for input into research projects without any warning, and managers who were reluctant to say no. So I didn't either.

Managers were in the office before me and left after me, making it harder for me to keep sensible hours myself. Sometimes and often without notice, I was required to work late—until nine, ten, or later—to meet a deadline.

This was partly because of my own inexperience. While I had reasonable data-analysis knowledge, I wasn't experienced at utilising the efficiency of the computer and spent longer trying to figure out what on earth I was doing than I do now. Using new data sets brought its own challenges because I had to research everything from scratch. Unfamiliar with the sector, I found this research even harder as I had to learn the subject matter too. A detail-oriented perfectionist, I was given the perfect rabbit warren to tumble into.

I was also isolated and rarely had anyone else to ask for help. Apart from one or two Excel gurus, nobody else had advanced knowledge of statistics, so when I was stumped, I was really stumped.

And frustrated.

I was dealing with a heavy workload, an inability to prioritise, and a tendency towards being overly detail orientated and perfectionistic—all in a fast-changing workplace. Such things were manageable when I felt I was working for a purpose, but words of encouragement or positive feedback were rare, and my motivation, energy, and enthusiasm were waning. I received plenty of constructive criticism, but without the positive feedback that motivates me so well. Cynicism and negativity pervaded the team, and I began to dread being in the office.

The event precipitating my depressive episode was my performance review. For the past six months, I felt I had gone above and beyond to do a good job, frequently working outside my comfort zone (which for me was extremely emotionally draining). I'd put a lot of myself—body, soul, and mind—into my work. But after being on the job for over eighteen months, I still achieved the same performance review. I felt as though I'd been kicked in the teeth.

My depression grew, and I began isolating myself. Talking to people became more tiring. I felt like I had to put on a mask to appear "normal." I felt I needed to hide the truth. Socialising made me feel physically uncomfortable, and meetings made me feel as though I was lying in a coffin, unable to break out.

Wearing negative-tinted spectacles; I interpreted every single event in the most personally damning way. I hated being at work, felt no sense of achievement or purpose, and felt trapped. I didn't feel clever enough to move on, and I didn't have the emotional energy for a new start.

I lacked energy and drive and sank lower and lower into my pit of despair.

Hence my crisis.

■ ■ ■

As part of my recovery, I realised I needed to work smarter rather than harder. I had already tried to work all the hours in the day, and then more, to no avail. The turning point was reading *Essentialism* by Greg McKeown (2014).

His principle is simple: do less, but do it better. In his book he discusses why prioritisation is so important and gives strategies for doing so.

It completely changed my outlook on life.

I realised I'd been addicted to being busy rather than effective. I could even be efficient, but I still wasn't effective. I realised I had to cut out all unnecessary activities (which I began to think of as my noise). I adopted his suggestion that if an opportunity wasn't a "hell yeah," then it was a no, no matter how beneficial it might appear.

I had already eliminated a lot of negativity by removing activities (and people) that didn't actively make me happy. Feeling I "should" do something was a massive red flag telling me I didn't really want to do whatever it was and that I needed to consider carefully whether I should actually do it. Thinking purposefully about whether I really wanted to see a friend, for example, either (a) convinced me I did actually want to see that friend or (b) helped me realise I needed to prioritise myself and spend the time nourishing myself instead, guilt-free. Either choice would be a win-win for both of us. I'm not great company if I'm not happy and/or don't want to be there! But despite cutting down on things I didn't want to do, I still had a lot of noise and not enough time to enjoy the happy times. So I started to identify, and then try to eliminate, my distractions one by one.

It was tough. Distractions can be fun, and they distract you because they interest you. I was scrolling through Facebook many times a day, but even after hiding neutral and negative people's posts, I still felt unsatisfied and incomplete after I'd done so. Reading the news on my mobile phone left me upset at the sadness in the world, and I was unable to find any happiness and joy in it.

So I changed the way I used technology. Initially, I turned off mobile data on my phone. I was simultaneously panicky at being adrift without an Internet connection and relieved that I wouldn't have to succumb to it. It was wonderful; by turning mobile data off, I wasn't able to mindlessly log on to the Internet without consciously being aware of what I was doing. I've since discovered there are apps such as Moment[28] that track your mobile usage and shut you out of your phone if you are on it for too long each day. I loved this unassuming but incredibly useful app—until I was at a dinner party and my phone

---

28 https://inthemoment.io/.

started screeching at me. I eventually turned the notifications off, but it's still extremely useful to see just how much time I'm spending on my phone, and I know I can turn those notifications on again if I need to.

As for the news, well, initially I felt extremely guilty for not tuning in to it. I didn't feel informed and felt I would be judged for admitting so. But because watching the news made my mental health so much worse, I had no choice but to stop.

Because I was prioritising positive mental health, I instead sought out other news sources promoting good news, such as the *Huffington Post*.[29] The Huffington Post's "Good News" section promotes stories that make you feel warm and fuzzy inside. Which makes me wonder why we are so addicted to the sensationalism of our current mainstream news stations, but that's another book…

I also tried to simplify everything I possibly could to make my life easier. I was excellent at creating purpose in my life (one of the factors for happiness), but I didn't have enough pleasure.[30] I was an errands master. Why wait for tomorrow when I could do it today? I created more work for myself by trying to do everything, and do it immediately. I'd been running around like a headless chicken, and now I'd completely forgotten where I'd left my head. So, to create more time for doing the things I love, I decided

---

29 http://www.huffingtonpost.com/good-news/.
30 Paul Dolan, *Happiness by Design: Change What You Do, Not How You Think* (United Kingdom: Penguin, 2014).

to try to reduce the number of errands I needed to do. I halved the time I spent cleaning our flat when I realised it didn't need to be clinically clean. I batched errands so that I did them quickly in one go rather than heading out numerous times a week to the same places.

While it might appear mundane,[31] the fact that I had five email addresses stressed me out. My inbox of horrors was multiplied by five every day. So I deleted three addresses, and life became slightly simpler.

I also simplified my finances. Upon taking stock, I realised I had accounts with three banks under two names.[32] One bank gave better service, interest rates, and mobile banking and had branches nearer to our flat, so it was an easy decision to close my accounts with the other two. Now banking is easy and quick, and I can easily see where my money is (or isn't). One fewer unnecessary headache.

In the spirit of tidying, I read Marie Kondo's book *Spark Joy*.[33] While I have always been a fan of tidying up and clearing out, much to my husband's dismay, I was rather overeager when throwing things out. He sometimes complained that if he stayed still long enough, he'd be thrown out too. Or that I was going to throw away so many things

---

31 I'm a firm believer that the little things can turn into the big things.

32 Completely legally, I hasten to add, having used both my maiden and married names.

33 Marie Kondo, *Spark Joy: An Illustrated Guide to the Japanese Art of Tidying: A simple, effective way to banish clutter forever* (London: Vermilion, 2014).

our flat would look like it had been burgled. Fortunately he isn't sentimental.

Kondo taught me a different approach. While she did advocate clearing the house of unwanted or useless clutter, she forced me to ask whether items sparked joy for us. If they did, we kept them. If they didn't, they were donated to the charity shop, recycled, or sold. Using this method, I saved a quilt I had made as a child. On the way to putting it in the recycle pile, I realised that the colours suited and brightened up our bedroom far better than the spare room, which was its original resting place. It wasn't that I needed to donate the quilt to charity but that it needed a new room instead where it could be displayed to its full potential. The quilt now makes me happy whenever I see it.

The overall result? Our flat contains only things we love or need and nothing else. My clothes are ones that I love, fit me, and flatter my body shape. Treasured mementos are in a small, beautiful box on top of our wardrobe. Our paperwork is a fraction of its original size, making it easier to find what we need. Our sofas no longer hide old canvases and picture frames behind them. Cleaning has become simpler, faster, and easier. Our flat is more peaceful, welcoming, and relaxing and an inspirational place for me to spend time in. Spending time in our newly joyful flat has made me realise just how much I didn't like spending time in it before. My sanctuary from the world now actually feels like a sanctuary and makes me happy.

Simplifying my life has made it easier to live in. I love spending time with family, friends and doing the things I enjoy—and the best bit? I now have time for all of it.

j. Prioritise Yourself

I was brilliant at prioritising—other people. I was sent to boarding school when I was eight years old and, despite my strongest attempts otherwise, stayed in the same school until I was eighteen. I'd originally agreed to go after reading many of Enid Blyton's *Malory Towers* and *St Clare's* books, but I found out too late that the reality wasn't like the books at all. I'd been conned.

After a bit of a turbulent start, I realised that life was easier if I was liked by my peers. This view may seem innocent enough, but it led to decades of prioritising other people's needs at the expense of my own. It fed my mental illness.

I felt I couldn't say no to people nor tell them if I didn't want to do something. I didn't want to upset them and so instead would reluctantly say yes. I found ways of disengaging and avoiding difficult conversations rather than simply tackling issues head on. I developed a wonderful ability to be passive aggressive. My polite and calm demeanour hid a turbulent and often very angry interior.

I tried to write or paint out my feelings, but these attempts were never successful enough, and I began to resent even those people closest to me. Awkward and unpredictable, my moods affected how I experienced life, and I felt trapped and constrained by other people's needs. It became so bad that at times I couldn't remember what *I* liked, I was so used to doing what I thought others wanted. I climbed Mount Kilimanjaro because I wanted to spend a week with friends. I never had the urge to climb the damn thing, and I'm sure I'll never climb it again! I wasn't strong enough to be my authentic self.

I felt I would frighten people away if I was honest and true about my feelings. My role was to look after others. I feared that if I let them into the darkest recesses of my soul, they'd find out what an awful person I was. They wouldn't like or love me anymore.

k. Talk to a Professional

Cognitive behavioural therapy (CBT) has generally been considered to be effective in treating depression.[34] *The National Institute for Health and Care Excellence (NICE) recommends CBT in certain situations,* [35] *and the National Health Service prescribes it to particular patients. However,*

---

34 David. F. Tolin, "Is Cognitive-Behavioral Therapy More Effective than Other Therapies? A Meta-Analytic Review," *Clinical Psychology Review* 30 (2010): 710–720, doi:10.1016/j.cpr.2010.05.003. http://www.sciencedirect.com/science/article/pii/S0272735810000899.

35 National Institute for Health and Care Excellence, "Depression in Adults: Recognition and Management," *NICE Guidelines* [CG90] (2009, last updated April 2016), https://www.nice.org.uk/guidance/cg90/

the evidence surrounding it is not without controversy, and recent studies have not been able to replicate the findings of previous research projects and meta-analyses.[36]

The Cochrane Common Mental Disorders Group is currently investigating the effects of CBT on a range of outcomes, such as quality of life and suicide prevention.[37] [38]

Other resources are available from:

- *The Centre for Clinical Interventions: http://www. cci.health.wa.gov.au/*
- *Psychology Tools: http://psychology.tools/*
- *Getselfhelp: http://www.getselfhelp.co.uk/index.html*
- *G. Butler and T. Hope,* Manage Your Mind: The Mental Fitness Guide *(1995)*

---

chapter/1-Guidance#treatment-choice-based-on-depression-subtypes-and-personal-characteristics.

36 Timothy. P. Baardseth, et al., "Cognitive-Behavioral Therapy versus Other Therapies: Redux," *Clinical Psychology Review* 33 (2013): 395–405, doi:10.1016/j.cpr.2013.01.004. http://www.sciencedirect.com/science/article/pii/S027273581300007X.

37 Christine Rummel-Kluge, Sandra Dietrich, and Nicole Koburger, "Behavioural and Cognitive-Behavioural Therapy Based Self-Help versus Treatment as Usual for Depression in Adults and Adolescents (Protocol)" *Cochrane Database of Systematic Reviews 2015, Issue 6* (2015), Art. No.: CD011744, doi: 10.1002/14651858.CD011744. http://onlinelibrary.wiley.com/doi/10.1002/14651858.CD011744/abstract.

38 V. Hunot, et al., "Cognitive Behavioural Therapies versus Treatment as Usual for Depression (Protocol)." *Cochrane Database of Systematic Reviews 2010, Issue 9* (2010), Art. No.: CD008699, doi: 10.1002/14651858.CD008699. http://onlinelibrary.wiley.com/doi/10.1002/14651858.CD008699/abstract.

I was signed off work and on the waiting list for cognitive behavioural therapy (again), but the wait for high-intensity support was nine long months. While I waited, I started working with a low-intensity therapist on my confidence, self-esteem, and assertiveness.

This particular self-guided therapy was amazing. I knew my self-esteem was low, but I had no idea just how low or how crippling it was. She led me, step by step, through the therapeutic process, and slowly but surely, life began to feel easier.

I learnt that I'd created weird and inflexible rules that I thought I had to live by. Yet they were crushing me and often completely inappropriate for the situation. I started to write down what I thought would happen and how I'd feel if I broke one of the rules, and then I'd deliberately break it to find out what did actually happen. It was fantastic! I had such fun breaking those debilitating and restrictive rules. No one else cared or even noticed; they were busy living their own lives.

It was liberating. I learnt that things nearly always turned out well, and if they didn't, well, that was OK too. I would cope. The world wasn't going to stop. I created far more freedom in my life and vowed to continue the experimentation. Plus it was just bloody good fun breaking all those bloody rules!

Assertiveness was another area of focus. I'd always struggled to be assertive. My upbringing had caused me to become extremely deferential to authority. As a perfectionist and someone who prefers to live by the rules, I was deferential to a fault and rarely—if ever—asserted my own needs. I wanted to please people, perfectly. But I was wrong.

Through my therapy, I learnt that I had the right to express my emotions. I had the right to change my mind. I had the right to say no. I had the right to say I needed thinking time. I had the right to make mistakes. I had the right to ask for what I wanted.

Therapy was transformative. During most of my childhood and all of my adult life, I hadn't believed I had any right to put myself first and acted as such. Doing so, I had accidentally and unintentionally reinforced my self-belief that I wasn't as worthy as other people. But now I learnt that I had the right to look after my own needs and prioritise myself.

I had started practising this by removing all the "shoulds" from my life and focusing on activities that made me happy. But assertiveness was a whole new ball game.

I learnt techniques and strategies. I practised. I wound up my husband, who eventually mentioned that perhaps I didn't need to be quite so assertive at home. So I redoubled my efforts when I went back to work. I stopped saying "sorry" to strangers on the street when I really meant "excuse me"—I stopped apologising for existing. I practised speaking in more direct ways. I was honest about how I felt and asked for what I wanted. I found the bosses at work and told them how I thought the organisation could be improved. And the surprising thing? I was met positively *every single time.* I made new connections with people across the organisation that I would not have necessarily talked to before. I gained more respect from my colleagues, who were appreciative of my honesty and integrity. I got work done faster because I was open about what I needed to do the job well, and I asked for help when I needed it.

Why was this so important? Because I was implicitly learning that I deserved to be heard and deserved to have my needs met, where appropriate. I was valued by my team. I was generating results on my projects. I helped others voice their own concerns and work more effectively. And life became easier in all aspects. No longer having to double-guess a reaction or ruminating over unsaid words, I felt more balanced and more secure as a person. I started to actually believe that my own needs deserved to be attended to just as much as other people's. My confidence grew, and I took on larger and more important tasks, both in and outside of work.

Instead of passively being a victim of my negative spiral of despair, I was slowly and carefully reversing that same spiral into one of increasing confidence and happiness. Every single time I asserted myself, I felt a rush of empowerment, pride, and joy. I felt as though the world was my oyster and that I could do anything. I started entering art competitions and getting through some of the rounds. I started harder pieces of work. I went on more training courses and met new friends. I was proactively driving my positive, virtuous spiral upwards.

I can't and wouldn't want to pretend that the journey—which is still ongoing—has been easy. There are moments when my positive resolve fades, and I'm harassed by negative demons, sitting on my shoulder, whispering to me about how terrible I am. But these episodes are shorter than before, and my rational mind kicks in earlier. I know if I give myself the opportunity to dwell on a negative event, the thoughts will make me sad, so instead I choose to limit my ruminations and either do something about them or forget them by distracting myself with something that makes me happy. Easier said than done, but I'm getting there. I treasure and celebrate every small, positive step I make.

I.   Don't Compare

I was a sucker for comparisons. No matter how hard I tried not to, I would always compare myself to other people. I could and would compare myself to anyone and everyone in an attempt to make myself feel better. If I felt I was doing better than they were, I felt smug. However, if I felt I was doing worse than they were—which was the vast majority of the time—I would descend into a spiral of self-loathing. No one was too high for me to compare myself to. I beat myself up for not being Mother Teresa. I beat myself up for not running the country. I beat myself up for not having been wildly successful in the City by my thirties and already retired. I beat myself up for not being a world-renowned artist. If I could beat myself up about something, I would.

Most damaging, though, was comparing myself to my colleagues. I looked at everyone else in my team and felt disappointed in myself that I hadn't been promoted to a higher position since I'd joined three years earlier. I had set for myself the unrealistic expectation that I should be climbing a rung on the career ladder every two years or less. Any longer than this, and I was failing. Not only was I failing—the devil on my shoulder was telling me I was a failure. I was unworthy. Unworthy of life. Sometimes the devil was louder than other times. Sometimes he could be argued with and sometimes not. Whenever I thought about my career failures, though, I felt resentful. I felt I should have been developed for promotion or even promoted. I didn't understand why I had failed or why I was "less" than others.

It took me a very long time to change this way of thinking, and I admit I'm not always there. Some days, when I'm feeling particularly weak or vulnerable, I'll slip into assuming that I'm not as good as others or that my worth is determined by where in the pecking order I am.

But I have to remind myself that that simply isn't true. I have friends and family and a wonderful husband who love me—regardless of my job. None of them care about what I do, they just want me to be healthy and happy and support me to be as such. They spend quality time with me outside of work and often don't even ask about how I spend my working day. It really doesn't matter to them.

Work isn't the be-all and end-all to me anymore. I work to live. I work to create an income that gives me freedom to paint what I love and to spend my time with loved ones doing activities I enjoy. I don't need a mansion, a fancy car, or a yacht. All I need is time to spend with my husband, money for a cup of tea and slice of cake, time to catch up with friends, and money to buy my canvases and paints. It's a bonus to have money to drive to the coast to camp, and it's a real treat to ski in Europe, but I don't need fancy dining, swanky cocktail bars, or a nonstop social life to feel happy. In fact, those things often make me feel worse!

I wouldn't have the patience to clean or maintain a mansion. I get seasick, so the yacht wouldn't be a good idea. I don't drink alcohol, so swanky cocktails are wasted on me. I'm often vegan (and hungry), so fancy dining really doesn't appeal. I prefer quantity over quality, and tiny morsels of food just aren't enough.

Instead, I try to crowd out all of the negativity with positivity. I just don't let my devil talk to me. When he starts chattering, I start talking back. In fact, I don't talk—I shout. In his face. I talk loudly and proudly and in detail about just how lucky I am with the way things are in my life. I am perfect—just as I am. I'm a human being who's trying her best in life, always learning, and that is enough. I'll say it again—the devil is hard of hearing. I am enough. Just as I am.

LIVE

LOVE YOURSELF

hated myself. I always had since I'd gone to boarding school. I don't know where this hatred came from exactly. It might have been a misguided reaction to perceived parental rejection, comments made by peers during an impressionable time in my life, or social conditioning through media stereotypes. Wherever it came from, my self-loathing grew as I did, knowing no limits.

At university, I gained a stone in weight in six weeks when my antidepressants increased my appetite. Unable to lose the weight, I hated my new body and self even more. Every time I looked in the mirror, I felt disgusted.

During the good times, I was OK. Sometimes I could even believe I was attractive and laughed and danced with the best of them. But as soon as I'd broken one of my self-imposed rules or interpreted a situation negatively, I was back to self-loathing. Rationally I knew that I was all right, but I *felt* ashamed of my body, mind, and soul. And then felt ashamed about feeling ashamed. The cycle continued.

m. Nourish Your Body

But I wanted to break this spiral of negativity. I would never have spoken to anyone else in the same way I spoke to myself. So concentrating on the positives rather than the negatives, I began to focus on my healthy body as being an incredible piece of machinery. I marvelled at its (potential) strength and ability to move. I started to go to the gym, initially using the cycling machines, and then started attending classes as my confidence and fitness grew. I learnt how to swing and use kettlebells. I dabbled with high-intensity interval training (HIIT), a particularly brutal form of exercise where I alternated intense bursts of exercise with a less intense period of recovery. I lifted dumbbells. I tried Pilates. I sweated, grunted, swore, and occasionally became extremely angry, but my body became healthier and happier.

Exercise gave me a feeling of accomplishment and purpose. Exercise released endorphins, meaning I left the gym feeling happy and relaxed. My body grew stronger. I developed muscles in my stomach that I never thought I'd see. My arm muscles could lift heavier weights and aerobics became easier.

As mentioned before, I was feeding my body with wholesome, nutritious food too. Eating homemade, predominantly plant-based foods, I tried to nourish my body inside and out. By doing this, not only was I treating my body as it deserved to be treated, but I was unconsciously reinforcing the message to myself that I deserved to look after and nourish myself.

I also tried mental-health techniques. When I realised I was talking negatively to myself, I proactively tried to think about something else, or reminded myself about how lucky I am that my body is healthy. Yes, I have a big bum, which sometimes makes finding well-fitting jeans difficult. But it gives me added cushioning when I sit down, powers my legs when I cycle, ski, or run, and I know my husband certainly appreciates it! So maybe it's not all bad…

n. Dress for You

Taking my arse as an example (I'm writing this book so I can), instead of viewing it as a problem, I decided to reframe it as a positive. I realised that I felt most fat and ugly when I wore a particular pair of jeans that cut into my sides and (unfairly) gave me a muffin top. If I wanted a muffin, I'd eat the bloody thing, not wear it. So I decided there was only one solution: go shopping. I donated my ill-fitting jeans to the charity shop and bought another pair that felt comfortable *and* flattered my body shape. The new jeans were a revelation. Instead of feeling crappy when I put them on, I now felt fabulous. I felt more confident walking down the street. I walked taller and held my head high. It was incredible—for a mere five pounds, I'd temporarily transformed not only my image but my self-confidence and self-esteem as well. A bargain for a fiver!

I cleared out any clothes that made me feel boring, fat, ugly, or insecure, and started replacing them (slowly) from the charity shop with flattering, well-fitting, comfortable clothes that I loved. I was frustrated that my wardrobe was dominated by black, so I deliberately chose gorgeous dresses in brighter colours to lift my mood. I changed my accessories so that conservative clothes were brightened up by quirky and unusual combinations of shoes or jewellery. And it was fun! I took photographs of my outfits and put them into my online journal with a note about how they had made me feel.

Not all outfits worked. One dress I'd optimistically bought from eBay turned out to be a tad too short for the office. I spent a very uncomfortable day pulling it down so that I didn't accidentally flash my knickers. But through the experience, I learnt I preferred knee-length skirts or dresses, and that dress was another lovely donation to the charity shop.

Over time I began to learn more about the clothing shapes that made me feel happier and more comfortable in my own skin. I learnt how to display my creativity and identity through the way I dressed and presented myself to the world. I felt I was projecting a more authentic image of myself and had gained the freedom to be my truest self. I felt liberated, happy, and confident. I felt like me.

o. Take Yourself on a Date

As an anxious and quiet child, I'd spent much of my time alone, writing, reading, drawing, and creating. But as I became older and gained a husband and active art career as well as a full-time job and friends, I had limited the time I spent alone to the absolute minimum.

But I still loved my quiet time. As an introvert, I'd learned the importance of using any available moments of peace and quiet as an opportunity to recharge and rest. And while I was very authentic to my husband, I didn't always feel comfortable doing exactly what I wanted when I was wish him, because I also wanted him to be happy. I wanted us to enjoy activities together.

As I started thinking, I realised I hadn't organised a day to hang out with myself by myself for months and months, possibly longer. In fact, it was so long ago, I had no idea what I wanted to do.

I considered seeing a musical, but I didn't have enough money for the ticket, so that idea was quickly discarded. I considered taking myself out for a meal, but eating at a restaurant alone has always daunted me, so I decided to start with small steps instead. As a fan of sofas, coffee, and cakes, I decided my special time would be to take myself out for a coffee.

Worried about being left alone with my thoughts for too long, I also took my own entertainment with me. I brought my book, journal, and lots of pens. It felt strange, taking myself on a date, but also strangely exciting. I didn't need anyone else to give me permission to do anything; I could choose—and do—exactly what I wanted. (Well, there were some limits, such as money. And the law.) I could spend as long as I liked making my way to the cafe, mooching in the shops, and gently pondering life. I could sit anywhere I wanted, do exactly as I wanted, and stay as long as I liked.

Those few hours were bliss. I pottered about, read, and wrote. The gift of time and solitude felt luxurious and made me feel calm, peaceful, and balanced. Again, I was reinforcing to myself that I deserved nourishing and nurturing—and all for the price of a coffee and cake.

p. Celebrate Your Successes

This was tough for me. I loved to set myself unachievably high targets and goals. And if I fell short, I felt I had failed. If I was complimented, I looked for unspoken criticisms. If things went well, I feared things would quickly change.

An important part of my recovery has been to learn to celebrate my successes. When I write in my journal at night, I list the things I'm proud of doing. And I'm not judging these things by where I was last year; I'm measuring them by where I am right now. Because that's all that matters.

When I returned to work after my illness, I was petrified. The last time I had physically come near the office, I ended up hyperventilating and crying. God only knew how I'd react to actually walking into the building and seeing people again. I didn't know how much they knew about my absence or how they would react to my return. I was scared.

So I set myself a realistic target of simply aiming to walk through the front door on that first day. It didn't matter what happened afterwards; all that counted was that I'd gotten inside the building.

It was tough. I wanted to run away. I wanted to enter the revolving door, walk a revolution, and then exit again. But I also knew that this was an important step in my recovery and that the only way of finding out whether I'd be OK was to give it a try. I could always leave if I needed to.

Fortunately I work with a lovely group of people, and yes, I did manage to walk into the building. And I rejoiced in that. I didn't care what I would have thought a year before. I didn't care what others thought about me. I was just pleased that I had made *my* small step forward. That was enough for the day. Anything else was a bonus. I had gotten into the building. And I was proud.

CONNECT

Humans are social creatures. The National Health Service (NHS) recommends we build "stronger, wider social connections" to help "feel happier and more secure, and give us a greater sense of purpose."[39] The Royal College of Psychiatrists recommends speaking to someone close to you about how you feel as "part of the mind's natural way of healing."[40]

It was a month into my sick leave, and I had been hiding away from the world. I once read that back in the days when we were cave people, if a child was in need, the child cried out to draw attention to itself. But if no one came, the child stopped crying and quietly hid in the cave for safety until someone did come. Doing this protected

39 NHS, "Connect for Mental Wellbeing," *Stress, Anxiety and Depression,* http://www.nhs.uk/conditions/stress-anxiety-depression/pages/connect-for-mental-wellbeing.aspx, last reviewed May 2016.

40 Royal College of Psychiatrists, "Depression," *Health Advice, Problems & Disorders* (June 2015), http://www.rcpsych.ac.uk/healthadvice/problemsdisorders/depression.aspx. Accessed 27.06.2016.

the child from predators, and this was what I had done, thousands of years later. I had retreated into my flat, hiding away from the world and all of its many threats. My depression was my body and mind's way of telling me that I needed some time out. I needed time to stop and reflect on my life and to give myself some self-care. For me, depression is a useful evolutionary mechanism that warns me when the way I'm living is unsustainable and when something needs to change. The worse the depression, the more urgent the need for change.

During my time off sick, I had cancelled all my plans and focused on spending quality time with my husband and myself. Often and easily tired, I took life at a slower pace and rested as much as I needed. The smallest tasks were exhausting, and I struggled in even the most mundane situations. My body needed time and rest to heal.

To give an example, my husband and I travelled to Central London to visit an art exhibition. Normally a savvy Londoner, I navigate the London Underground warren confidently and quickly, without a flinch or pause. But the sicker version of myself hated it. Couldn't bear being close to other human beings. Hated the noise. Felt every single irate word or stressed retort (to someone else) as though it was directed at me. I picked up and took on other people's stresses and complaints as though they were my own.

I was unable to book train tickets, navigate the ticket barrier, or even look after my own safety. I forgot to put my debit card away at Leicester Square station and had to be gently reminded by my husband, lest I be pickpocketed.

Would it have been pickpocketing if someone had taken the card directly out of my hand? Did the item have to be in a pocket or bag? Would it have been robbery? Opportunism? My own fault?

It wasn't just strangers I struggled with. I couldn't look into people's eyes, not even those of close friends or family. I wasn't brave enough to look into their souls, and I was terrified of what they might find in mine. I didn't want them to see my pain, my suffering. I felt unmasked, vulnerable, and unsure; my world stood on quicksand and I was sinking.

Socialising was out of the question. Physically uncomfortable and socially awkward, I found that it was one step too far for me. We had cancelled all our plans, explaining I wasn't well. When I'm depressed, my relationships seriously suffer as I withdraw into my own chaotic mind and isolate myself.

So now, one month after retreating into my cave, I was starting to come out of it. It would take many months before I felt more firmly balanced, and even a year on, I would still struggle with certain types of socialising, but this one-month turning point was important. I started to— and most importantly, wanted to—connect with people.

I had realised that I much prefer socialising with small numbers of people and having the opportunity for quality conversations. Large groups in unfamiliar surroundings with loud sounds were appalling to my fragile mind. So I started to socialise in the best way I knew how.

I started by meeting a close friend in Kensington. I hadn't seen her for months, nor had I travelled by myself in central London for weeks, so this was a big step for my poorly mind. I found it difficult to be around strangers on the train, and the unnerving hustle and bustle around the shops put me on edge. But I also wanted to get better, and socialising was an important part of my recovery. And she is such an important person to me.

I was very lucky. She showed me the beautiful Kensington Roof Gardens and then led me to a gorgeous tea shop for delicious cake and tea. As you know by now, I love cake! I appreciated exploring somewhere new and loved sitting with her, catching up and watching the world go by. Even though it had been difficult venturing out alone and I had wanted to turn back numerous times during my journey there, I was extremely glad that I hadn't and that I had gone through with it. I left feeling warm and fuzzy inside. And elated that I had managed to do it.

Seeing my friend set a positive trajectory for the rest of my recovery and the ongoing maintenance of my positive mental health. I now don't commit to too many social engagements and prioritise those where I know I'll have the best-quality conversations. I carefully consider the venue and whether it's going to be challenging or not to me. The more challenging the venue, the more uncomfortable, exhausted, and self-critical I'll be. If there's a special reason I might want to go somewhere, but the venue is difficult, I'll decide whether I'm up to it. I'm keen to challenge myself, and the best way of learning if I'm up for something is to just give it a try. Yet at the same time, I need to make sure I don't put myself in particularly difficult or destructive situations. It's a constant balancing act.

Prioritising social engagements has been key. Living in London, I've sometimes been invited to three events on the same night. Previously I'd try to make them all, going from one to the next and then the next. But constantly clock-watching isn't enjoyable, and I suffered constant guilt for being late or leaving early. Definitely unnecessarily stressful. Instead, I now commit to one, possibly two, invitations a week. The rest of the time, I have alone time, painting time, or quality time with my husband. I've found through trial and error that socialising this amount is the right balance for me: less than this, and I'd jeopardise my friendships and get cabin fever; any more, and I'd start to tire and crave my solitude and even begin to resent having to leave my home.

Now I look forward to seeing my friends. I know I'll feel better having met with them and leave with that connected, happy feeling inside. I have more energy and can concentrate better when listening to them. My memory has improved, and I better remember what they've actually said.

I also try to practise mindfulness, really experiencing and appreciating the time we have together rather than worrying about my next task or appointment. Previously I wasn't really ever present with them; my mind was elsewhere, rocketing from one to-do list to the next, worrying about the future, and beating myself up about the past. Now I try to give my friends my undivided, full attention and actively listen to them. Friendships have flourished.

Friends have also responded very positively to my openness and honesty. Talking to people about my insecurities and vulnerabilities has fostered a sharing environment where they feel free to talk as well. Sharing our authentic selves has allowed acceptance to thrive and mutual support to grow. No need for a front at all: I am loved and accepted just as I am. As my dad told me recently, I am loved *because* of my imperfections. I am perfectly imperfect.

And at the end of the day, social niceties are important but not the be-all and end-all. It's far more important to be our authentic and honest selves. I am reminded of something a friend said recently. When I left a country fair because I felt unable to make any more polite conversation, he suggested perhaps I should make impolite conversation.

Now that sounds like it could be fun!

EXPLORE

q. Discover Nature

There is an increasing amount of research suggesting that being in natural surroundings can help with stress,[41] depression,[42] anxiety,[43][44] and mental health generally.[45][46][47]

---

41 C. W. Thompson, et al., "More Green Space Is Linked to Less Stress in Deprived Communities: Evidence from Salivary Cortisol Patterns," *Landscape Urban Plann.* 105 (2012): 221–229, doi:10.1016/j. landurbplan.2011.12.015.

42 M. G. Berman, et al., "Interacting with Nature Improves Cognition and Affect for Individuals with Depression," *J. Affect. Disord.* 140 (2012): 300–305, doi:10.1016/j.jad.2012.03.012.

43 K. M. M. Beyer, et al., "Exposure to Neighbourhood Green Space and Mental Health: Evidence from the Survey of the Health of Wisconsin," *Int. J. Environ. Res. Public Health* 11 (2014): 3453–3472, doi:10.3390/ijerph110303453.

44 G. Bratman, et al., "The Benefits of Nature Experience: Improved Affect and Cognition," *Landscape and Urban Planning* 138 (2015): 41–50.

45 D. G. Pearson and T. Craig, "The Great Outdoors? Exploring the Mental Health Benefits of Natural Environments," *Front. Psychol.* 5, no. 1178 (2014), doi: 10.3389/fpsyg.2014.01178.

46 I. Alcock, et al., "Longitudinal Effects on Mental Health of Moving to Greener and Less Green Urban Areas," *Environ. Sci. Technol.* 48 (2014): 1247–1255, doi:10.1021/es403688w.

47 G. Bratman, et al., "Nature Experience Reduces Rumination and Subgenual Prefrontal Cortex Activation," *PNAS* 112, no. 28 (2015): http://www.pnas.org/content/112/28/8567.abstract.

My husband and I have always enjoyed exploring the outdoors. Well, he's always loved it, and I've learned to love it more with him. Together we have walked and ice-climbed around Snowdonia and camped our way around Spain. When exploring without him, I've walked the Inca Trail and climbed Mount Kilimanjaro and Mount Kinabalu after I mistakenly left a close friend in charge of the agendas. I realised when climbing Kilimanjaro that I'd do anything to spend holiday time with this friend—even climbing nearly six thousand metres. (Although that won't be happening again!)

I've always loved spending time by the sea and in mountains. Having spent many childhood holidays in Northern Ireland, I have fond memories of those summer days on the beach. And as a keen skier, I dash to the mountains whenever possible. I find that being around the sea or in the mountains gives me a sense of awe, peace, and perspective that I simply cannot find elsewhere. The vastness of the ocean and the dramatic, inhospitable heights of mountains remind me that problems I am ruminating on will most likely turn out OK and that we are each one tiny part of an incredible planet.

Living in London can be difficult. The traffic, pollution, and number of people make it hard to connect with Mother Earth. It's hard to see the stars, and I rarely hear birds sing. Fortunately, London has a large number of parks, meaning green space is never far away. We picnic on the grass as the sun sets, overlooking the city's iconic skyline. We laze around reading books during hot summer afternoons. We walk along green trails within our hectic city.

And we also escape the city. There are numerous country walks a short train ride away from London that are well marked and easy to navigate. *Time Out* even produces a book of recommended walks that includes maps, directions, and train timetables from London along with suggested lunching spots.

So last summer, during my recovery, we walked as far as we could, up hills and down dales. And with every step, my mind continued to mend. I was able to consider what had gone wrong and why I had burnt out. I pondered my quality of life, my daily habits, and that ever-elusive work-life balance. I discussed various ideas with my husband and asked him to challenge my negative assumptions and fears. I confided in him when I was riddled with anxiety, and he helpfully told me when my fears were reasonable and when they weren't. He helped me to realise my fears weren't reasonable most of the time. On the rare instances where they were reasonable, we brainstormed potential solutions together.

We camped for four days in Yorkshire and walked and walked and walked. We had paused our lives and taken time out to heal. We returned to our roots, focusing only on where we were going to walk, where and when we were going to eat, and where we were going to sleep. Life was simple and beautiful.

It wasn't always comfortable; with night-time temperatures around zero, we had to cuddle close, but the simplicity of our worries was a welcomed change and helped us to connect with ourselves and each other. We were unconnected to the Internet, rarely had a telephone signal, and were finally able to gain perspective over our lives at home, helped by the distance we had travelled.

As we returned to London and my life returned to a sense of normality, we kept our habit of being in nature as much as possible. I brought flowers and plants into our flat. We continued to explore country walks outside London on weekends. We continued to ski and started training more regularly in Milton Keynes and farther afield. We took walks along the river and mindfully appreciated the moment instead of rushing through it.

And this has continued ever since. While this winter brought its own challenges due to the cold and rain, we still went walking whenever we could and spent more time skiing in the mountains. We've learnt that living in London can be wonderful but that it's also important to escape it now and again to regain perspective. Perspective is key.

r. Learn Something New

The New Economics Foundation (NEF) has developed five evidence-based actions to improve well-being. One of these is to learn. Learning is linked with "positive effects on well-being, reports of life satisfaction, optimism and efficacy" for adults.[48]

48 J. Aked, et al., "Five Ways to Wellbeing," accessed May 21, 2016, http://b.3cdn.net/nefoundation/8984c5089d5c2285ee_t4m6bhqq5.pdf.

Learning a new skill is underrated. It gives a sense of purpose, is interesting, an opportunity to meet new people, and results in the satisfaction of achievement. Knowing this, while I was recovering and when I felt up to it, I decided to try out some new things with varying levels of scariness.

First on my list was to make new arty friends in London. I looked on Meetup.com for, well, an arty meet-up and was spoilt for choice. So many different options all over London. But I also knew that if the meet-up was far away from home, I would be more reluctant to go and could potentially find the whole experience too tiring and overwhelming. So I decided on a local group—and it was brilliant!

I loved the Sunday morning and afternoon drawing sessions on the Southbank, which were very affordable with just the right amount of tuition. Learning the hard way that perhaps I shouldn't try to do both sessions in one day (I was seeing double and completely exhausted by the end), I nevertheless continued on and developed my drawing practice as a result.

But while it was a brilliant experience and great for developing my skills, I didn't strongly connect with anyone there on a personal level, and so I continued on my quest, knowing I could return to the Sunday sessions as and when I wanted to.

Next on my list was learning how to boulder. Well, actually it was on my husband's list, but I thought it could be rather cool. I had images of myself looking gorgeously toned and muscly, dancing up daunting and impossible walls, clinging on to them like a long-legged spider.

The reality wasn't quite like that. I have short legs. I am neither flexible nor strong. My imagination was abruptly brought back to reality with a hard thud. It was great to support my (legally blind) husband to help him do something he loves, and I certainly enjoyed the physical-exercise aspect of it, but I wasn't passionate enough about it to continue doing it on a regular basis. My time was precious, and for my own mental health, I had to prioritise the ways in which I used it.

The third and most successful thing I tried was a language—Spanish. I've always loved Spanish-speaking countries and have wanted to master the language for years. This desire started nearly a decade ago during a brief stint in Central and South America and has lasted ever since. I had heard about an app called Duolingo,[49] which is both free and fun to use, and so I decided to give it a go. After all, what did I have to lose?

I will say it straight out: I love Duolingo. I hadn't realised that learning could be so interactive and suited to a busy lifestyle. I could do bite-sized lessons regularly to consolidate what I already knew and progress on to more difficult words. It felt game-like, with targets and goals, and I responded very positively to its encouragement. I

---

49 https://www.duolingo.com/.

was able to practise my pronunciation in the safety and privacy of my flat, and my confidence in speaking grew.

It was the most successful way I've learnt a language to date—and also so fun!

So having tried all this, what did I learn about learning?

i)   Enjoy the process. It won't be half as fun if you approach it with a fixed mind-set or obsess about your flaws. Embrace a growth mind-set[50] and enjoy making mistakes as you learn.

ii) Be curious. There are a million different things to try out there.

iii) Go with an open mind. Getting out of your comfort zone in a constructive way can help build confidence and self-esteem. You never know what might happen.

iv) Don't be afraid to stop. While some learning experiences can be great, others may not spark your passion or be quite right for you, so if it's not working out, don't force it. Appreciate, though, that any type of learning is going to have ups and downs and establish whether the difficulties are part of the overall learning process or whether you're just not that interested in the activity.

v)   Prioritise. The main limit is your time, so use it wisely.

---

50 Carol Dweck, *Mindset: How You Can Fulfil Your Potential* (United States: Ballantine Books, 2008).

FEED YOUR SOUL

s. Draw

Some research has shown that there is a correlation between art therapy and detecting or improving depression.[51][52]

I was unable to leave the house for more than two or three hours a day. I had cancelled all inessential activities and was prioritising activities that made me happier.

One of these activities was art. I have always drawn. Older members of my family were professional artists, and I grew up surrounded by portraits. I drew and painted throughout my childhood years and as a young adult sought out opportunities to develop my skills. It was

51 G. Bar-Sela, et al., "Art Therapy Improved Depression and Influenced Fatigue Levels in Cancer Patients on Chemotherapy," *Journal of Psycho-Oncology* 16 (2007): 980–984.

52 J. Wallace, et al., "The Use of Art Therapy to Detect Depression and Post-traumatic Stress Disorder in Pediatric and Young Adult Renal Transplant Recipients," *Pediatric Transplantation* 8, no. 1 (February 2004): 52–59, doi:10.1046/j.1397-3142.2003.00124.x.

therefore unsurprising that during a time of such emotional despair, I returned to art to soothe and nourish my soul.

When I was able to leave the house, my husband and I visited art exhibitions. Fortunately, living in London meant we were spoilt for choice and that the quality of work was extremely high. I had just enough energy to travel to Central London, view an exhibition, and then return home. On a good day, I could also fit in a coffee and a slice of cake. I learnt from the masters and was inspired by more recent works. I was energised by different artistic perspectives and soothed by different colours. I lost myself—and my sadness—in art.

It wasn't always easy to leave the flat. It took horrible amounts of energy, and I did occasionally have to interact with other people. But when I returned, I painted. And painted and painted. And painted some more. No matter what was happening outside, my flat was my sanctuary; specifically, my studio was my sanctuary. When painting, I lost all of my anxieties, my insecurities, and my sadness. All I could focus on was the relaxing and therapeutic action of applying paint to canvas. Commissioned to paint two zebras, I lost myself in those stripes. My detail-orientated brain obsessed over the blacks and whites until they were just right. I reworked and reworked and reworked the paint, and as I did, my subconscious mind started to process all that had happened and carried on healing. I felt serene, calm, and like a better, healthier, happier version of myself. There was no conflict, no stress, and no unhappiness, only joy.

I didn't always find painting easy. Some days it felt as though nothing went well, and I felt frustrated and angry. But I learnt during this time that if I persevered for long enough, I'd come out the other side with a painting I was proud of. I learnt to enjoy the process, to be mindful and present in every brushstroke. It was the closest to meditation I could get.

I often get told by people that they "can't" draw or that they're not creative enough. I believe that's rubbish. There's no innate talent in drawing; it's about learning and practising, just as apprentices did during the Renaissance. The reason I can paint the way I do is because I've practised for years and years, taught myself from others, and sacrificed time with friends and family so that I could practise my craft.

However, for those who still lack confidence, a new type of book has gained popularity recently that might reduce the fear of drawing. Mindfulness colouring books (for both adults and children) offer everyone the opportunity to enjoy the process of drawing. Guided through gorgeous designs, the drawer can choose whichever colours they want and become immersed in the healing process of drawing. Even my husband has been converted (and I've appreciated having a more relaxed version of him around the flat!)

t. Make Music

I was walking down the main street in Peckham, about five weeks into my recovery. It was a busy day, but the sun was shining and the weather was warm. And I wanted to sing.

This stopped me in my tracks. Because in that one split second, I realised I *hadn't* wanted to sing for months. And the urge to sing is one of my indicators of happiness. Since the start of the year, I'd been so stressed and focused on the mundane minutiae of life that singing was the last thing on my mind. I'd been miserable and silent—until now.

Beaming, I told my husband, who immediately understood the significance of this. I had just taken another solid step forward in my recovery: I now wanted to sing.

So I sang. In the shower, to the cats, in the car. I sang as I cycled—it is a very effective bicycle bell! I didn't care what I sounded like or if I even knew the words; I just wanted to make music and enjoy the experience.

I created happy playlists and listened to them over and over again. I listened to new music and avoided any songs that I associated with sadness or depression. As I sang, I also danced. I danced in the shower, in the living room, in the bedroom. I danced while I cooked and while I dressed.

Overall, I've learnt that it doesn't matter what you create or how you create it but only that you do something that nourishes your soul on a regular basis. Find a way of expressing how you feel in whichever way works for you. It could be anything; writing, drawing, singing, writing comedy, making miniature cars out of tin cans - anything. Protect and cherish that thing with your life. Nothing is more important than your health.

WORK

I decided to dedicate a section of this book to work because (a) work was the main factor that triggered my last depressive episode, and (b) as we spend so much time at work, it's vital that we find balance and are happy and healthy there. Some of the resources below discuss stress rather than depression, but as depression and stress can be very interlinked, and as these resources are also helpful, they have been included.

The British Occupational Health Research Foundation has helpfully summarised the available evidence around mental health in the workplace in "Workplace Interventions for People with Common Mental Health Problems: Evidence Review and Recommendations" (2005). It states that:

- *For employees who have not developed mental-health problems, stress-management techniques can be helpful to both themselves and their organisation. Using more than one method or technique was more beneficial than using a single technique.*

- *For those employees who were at risk, it found strong evidence that an individual approach (rather than an organisational approach) was more effective in managing common mental-health problems.*
- *And for those employees who were already experiencing common mental-health problems in their workplace, there was strong evidence in favour of individual therapy, especially cognitive behavioural therapy.*[53]

The Cochrane Work Group has analysed the effects of interventions to help depressed people at work. It found that in addition to regular treatment, "changes at work such as work modification or coaching...reduced sickness absence to a moderate extent." Cognitive behavioural therapy [54]*(online or telephone based) also "reduced sickness absence to a moderate extent."*

---

53 British Occupational Health Research Foundation, "Workplace Interventions for People with Common Mental Health Problems: Evidence Review and Recommendations," September 2005, http://www.bohrf.org.uk/downloads/cmh_rev.pdf.

54 Karen Nieuwenhuijsen, et. al., "Interventions to Improve Return to Work in Depressed People," *Cochrane Database of Systematic Reviews 2014, Issue 12* (December 2014), Art. No.: CD006237, doi: 10.1002/14651858.CD006237.pub3. http://www.cochrane.org/CD006237/OCCHEALTH_interventions-to-help-depressed-people-resume-work. Accessed 27.06.2016.

Moving away from the medical perspective, the Health and Safety Executive is "the national independent watchdog for work-related health, safety and illness. It acts in the public interest to reduce work-related death and serious injury across Great Britain's workplaces."[55] It has a large number of resources on its website and has published a useful report titled "Best practice in rehabilitating employees following absence due to work-related stress." This report lays out tangible, practical ways that organisations—of varying sizes—can support employees to return to and remain in work.[56]

The CIPD is "the professional body for HR and people development."[57] Its website contains a wealth of information, and its "Mental Health in the Workplace" factsheet provides a useful summary of what mental health is and how to support employees' mental health at work.[58] It also provides a resource targeted for managers: "Developing

---

55 GOV.UK, https://www.gov.uk/government/organisations/health-and-safety-executive. Accessed 01.07.2016.

56 Institute for Employment Studies, "Best Practice in Rehabilitating Employees Following Absence Due to Work-Related Stress" for the Health and Safety Executive," (2003). http://www.hse.gov.uk/research/rrpdf/rr138.pdf.

57 CIPD, "About Us," accessed 2016. https://www.cipd.co.uk/cipd-hr-profession/about-us/.

58 CIPD, "Mental Health in the Workplace" Factsheet, (revised November 2015), https://www.cipd.co.uk/hr-resources/factsheets/mental-health-workplace.aspx#link_2.

Managers to Manage Sustainable Employee Engagement, Health and Well-Being."[59] *This detailed and informed publication articulates the best ways for managers to develop to effectively support their employees.*

---

59 CIPD, IOSH, and Affinity, "Developing Managers to Manage Sustainable Employee Engagement, Health and Well-Being," *Research Insight*, (November 2014), page 34. https://www.cipd.co.uk/binaries/developing-managers_2014.pdf.

TALK

The "Growing the Health and Well-Being Agenda: From First Steps to Full Potential" report by CIPD notes that open communication is crucial for personal and organisational well-being.[60]

I'd been in my role for nearly two years when my crisis hit. As my negative thoughts increased in severity and frequency, I began to see everything through negativity-tinted spectacles. Any situation was given the most negative interpretation possible, and I ruminated on my weaknesses constantly.

I also felt angry and unfairly treated. As I became more and more ill, I retreated into myself and resented being around anyone. I struggled to concentrate, my motivation disappeared, and I disengaged from work.

---

60 CIPD, "Growing the Health and Well-Being Agenda: From First Steps to Full Potential" policy report (January 2016), https://www.cipd.co.uk/binaries/health-well-being-agenda_2016-first-steps-full-potential.pdf.

One Wednesday morning I came into work. I'd noticed I had become more emotional in recent weeks and months, but on this Wednesday, I felt uncontrollably weepy for no apparent reason. I walked into the office and immediately had to dash to the loo. I couldn't stop crying.

I didn't know what had set me off or why this outburst was happening now. I felt at the whim of my body, and my emotions felt out of control. I realised I needed help.

u. Ask for Help

You can ask for support from your human resources department and also from the government's Access to Work scheme if you work in England. You may be offered an occupational health assessment and potentially be supported by an occupational rehabilitation consultant (provided by the government) to return to and stay in work.

Another helpful resource is the Mental Health & Employment: Helping People to Stay in Employment Toolkit for Individuals (2012),[61] which features many practical ideas for both employer and employee for improving mental health in the workplace. This toolkit contains a large number of additional resources and signposting to other organisations.

---

61 Published by the European Union Programme for Employment and Social Solidarity: http://base-uk.org/sites/base-uk.org/files/%5Buser-raw%5D/12-04/toolkit_individuals.pdf.

I contacted HR immediately and met with them later that day. I was completely honest for the first time. I had a history of depressive episodes and feared I was in the midst of another. I felt out of control and helpless and didn't know what to do.

Fortunately HR did. They supported me to tell my line manager and suggested that I specify the help I needed from her and also tell her what I'd commit to doing myself, such as seeing my GP. Communicating with my manager was wonderful. She responded in such a helpful and supportive way, and it felt as though a huge burden of secrecy had been lifted. Together, we started to navigate the support available.

v. Prioritise

The CIPD discusses individual-level barriers to positive behaviour for managers and offers solutions as to how these might be overcome. While "Developing Managers to Manage Sustainable Employee Engagement, Health and Well-Being" has been written specifically for those in management positions, this table contains very helpful information for all employees. One of its (many) recommendations for a challenging workload is to prioritise.[62]

---

62 CIPD, IOSH, and Affinity, "Developing Managers to Manage Sustainable Employee Engagement, Health and Well-Being," *Research Insight*, (November 2014), page 34. https://www.cipd.co.uk/binaries/developing-managers_2014.pdf

Essentialism *by Greg McKeown also describes techniques to learn how and what to prioritise.*[63]

It was brilliant to be honest about how I'd really been feeling. The professional mask I wore at work came off, and I felt I could be true to who I was. I was able to speak openly without fear of being perceived as weak, inadequate, or unprofessional. I was able to have constructive conversations, particularly when it came to workload.

Workload had always been problematic. Working in a frenetic and fast-paced organisation has always been a challenge for my introverted, perfectionist self. I hadn't wanted to seem incapable or unable to do my job, and so I had hidden my emotions and difficulties and tried to appear to be coping. Except that I wasn't.

Once I accepted that I could now be true to how I felt, my conversations with my manager improved significantly. Instead of hiding when I felt the pinch, I now actively flagged it, and together we brainstormed potential ways forward. I highlighted times when I anticipated a difficult task and/or heavy workload, and flagging when I was nervous about starting a new project meant we could have conversations about whether I needed additional support, training, or resources.

Speaking up when I felt the pressure also meant that my line manager had more of a realistic idea about how

---

63 Greg McKeown, *Essentialism: The Disciplined Pursuit of Less* (United Kingdom: Virgin Books, 2014).

long tasks took and was therefore able to support me better. She deprioritised other tasks that I needed to do, asked colleagues to help out where necessary, extended deadlines, and communicated sensible and realistic expectations to the rest of the organisation.

But most importantly, by speaking honestly and openly with her, I felt we were back on the same team again. I felt valued and protected.

FOCUS

w. Reduce Distractions

While we all need varying levels of stimulation in order to work at our optimum, distractions impair our memory and short-term attention[64] and affect our concentration.[65]

By speaking to my manager openly about my workload and what I was going to be doing when, I didn't have to worry about constantly being available to colleagues. I have always found trying to be "on call" extremely distracting. I am unable to become absorbed in serious or demanding tasks, and I struggle to achieve the sense of satisfaction that comes with productive and focused work. As an introvert, a lack of quiet and undisturbed

---

64 Susan Cain, *Quiet: The Power of Introverts in a World That Can't Stop Talking* (2012).

65 S. P. Banbury and D. C. Berry, "Office Noise and Employee Concentration: Identifying Causes of Disruption and Potential Improvements," *Ergonomics* 48, no. 1 (2005). http://www.tandfonline.com/doi/abs/10.1080/00140130412331311390.

concentration time makes me miserable. Something had to change.

My manager knew the projects I was working on, and we agreed I would check emails a maximum of once or twice a day. If she needed something urgently from me, she would speak to me or telephone me if I was working elsewhere. I didn't have to continually monitor Outlook, fearing what might arrive.

Actually I didn't want to think about Outlook at all. So I proactively reduced how frequently it disturbed my concentration. I turned off email notifications, meaning that I could work without being distracted by boxes popping up in the corner of my screen. I also turned off all notifications on my mobile apart from text messages, meaning I wasn't tempted to check my emails there either.

I changed Outlook so that it opened automatically on the calendar rather than my inbox. This was a revelation. Now when I had to check where a meeting was, I wasn't bombarded with urgent-looking emails demanding my immediate attention.

I changed my email view so that I saw only the title and author of the email rather than the email content as well. Again, this meant that I could engage with the email when I chose to rather than Outlook dictating where and how I spent my attention.

I also started using the tasks function in Outlook to capture everything I needed to do, setting reminders as required. I now had one single to-do list, organised by due date and priority, rather than numerous lists in numerous places. If I needed to do something, it went on my task list. And remember that I did only what was vital for my role; the principles of essentialism here were crucial. Nothing was allowed on my to-do list that wasn't essential. I had finally created space and time to do my job properly.

I didn't sign into our organisation's messenger service and stopped it from turning on automatically. I switched it on when I wanted to use it rather than allowing it to control me. I slowly but surely started to feel more in control of my work environment, to-do list, and workload.

x. Concentrate on a Single Task

We just cannot multi-task. What we believe is multi-tasking is actually doing a lot of separate tasks, one after the other. Multi-tasking makes us more likely to make mistakes and will also make our work take longer (Medina, 2008).[66]

Protecting concentration time was vital. I get a huge amount of satisfaction from doing a job well. I had noticed that when I tried to multitask and focus on numerous activities at once, my mind became muddled, forgetful, and far more stressed. I had spent the past eighteen months feeling harassed and unsatisfied, feeling I was doing

---

66 John Medina, *Brain Rules: 12 Principles for Surviving and Thriving at Work, Home and School* (Seattle: Pear Press, 2008).

many things simultaneously but not achieving as much as I expected to. So as part of my recovery, I rejected the idea that I could multitask and focused on single-tasking instead.

Contrary to what I anticipated, my productivity increased. With no distractions and the ability to focus on one activity at a time, I did each activity to a higher standard and faster. My memory improved, and I dropped fewer balls. I deliberately diarised blocks of time to work from home to focus on the most important tasks, undisturbed by colleagues walking past my desk.

By keeping a note of my most and least attentive times during the day, I learnt when I was most productive and saved the most challenging or important tasks for then. Instead of trying to force my mind and body to focus when it was in its daily mid-afternoon slump, I used that time to do less-challenging administrative work. My body and mind started to work together, rather than trying to work independently of each other.

I also continued to prioritise, setting myself one clear goal every day. I allowed myself the time to really focus on that one task and considered anything else I accomplished to be a bonus. Again, I had presumed that my productivity would decrease after taking this approach, but the opposite happened. Because I was taking the time to really think through a single issue, I explored it from more angles, stopped potential problems from developing, thought through the next actions in more detail, and communicated with colleagues more effectively as a result. So what happened overall? Large projects moved forward faster and to a higher standard, and I felt motivated, engaged with my work, and satisfied that I was achieving something meaningful every single day. Quite a change from a few months before.

SET UP YOUR WORKING ENVIRONMENT

Tim Lister and Tom DeMarco identified that the work-place was an important factor in their research three decades ago.[67] More important than the salary, experience, or time spent on the task was the amount of "privacy, personal space, control over their physical environments, and freedom from interruption" the workers had. In fact, open-plan offices "have been found to reduce productivity and impair memory. They're associated with high staff turnover. They make people sick, hostile, unmotivated, and insecure. Open-plan workers are more likely to suffer from high blood pressure and elevated stress levels... They're often subject to loud and uncontrollable noise, which raises heart rates; releases cortisol, the body's fight-or-flight 'stress' hormone; and makes people socially

---

67 Tim Lister and Tom DeMarco, "Programmer Performance and the Effects of the Workplace," *Proceedings of the 8th International Conference on Software Engineering*, IEEE Computer Society, 1985.

distant, quick to anger, aggress, and slow to help others" *(Cain, 2012).*[68]

This issue has been explored in depth since, and Croon et al. provide a helpful literature review in "The Effect of Office Concepts on Worker Health and Performance: A Systematic Review of the Literature." They summarise "that there is strong evidence that working in open workplaces reduces privacy and job satisfaction. Limited evidence is available that working in open workplaces intensifies cognitive workload and worsens interpersonal relations; close distance between workstations intensifies cognitive workload and reduces privacy; and desk-sharing improves communication" (De Croon, et al., 2005).[69]

I felt very lucky. My organisation had an agile working policy, meaning that we could work wherever we wanted to as long as we shared our location in our diary and were contactable. We could also work the hours we wanted as long as we worked our contracted and core hours every day. Assessed by outcomes, we had the freedom to determine how and where we worked the best.

---

68 Susan Cain, *Quiet: The Power of Introverts in a World That Can't Stop Talking* (2015), 84.

69 Einar M. De Croon, Judith K. Sluiter, P. Paul, F. M. Kuijer, and Monique H. W. Frings-Dresen, "The Effect of Office Concepts on Worker Health and Performance: A Systematic Review of the Literature," *Ergonomics* 48, no. 2: 119–134, 10 February 2005, http://senate.ucsf. edu/2013-2014/mb6-de%20croon%20ergonomics%20article%20 on%20workplace%20design.pdf.

I had a few issues though. If I had to work my contracted hours as a minimum, then the only variation could be an increase in hours. And working from home more meant it was dangerously easy for me to slip into longer working hours accidentally.

As someone who wanted to follow the rules, I was also unfortunately susceptible to presenteeism. Faced with a manager who was usually in the office earlier in the morning and later in the evening than I was, I felt as though I was underperforming constantly. She reassured me that I was doing fine and that she preferred working those hours, but her actions spoke louder than words, and it was extremely difficult to do anything else without feeling horribly guilty.

I felt I had to be always available to prove I was working, no matter where I was actually working that day. Nothing seemed to reassure me, and the constant worry and stress wore me into the ground.

After my crisis, I realised that I had to take control of my working environment rather than having it control me. The organisation had created their agile working policy to provide more flexibility and improve working conditions for colleagues, so why was I using it to beat myself up? I decided to make changes.

When I returned to work, I was very clear about how and where I was going to work. Working from home two to three days a week was the perfect balance for me, combining social interaction at the office and quiet, focused concentration time at home. I kept meetings for Tuesdays and Thursdays where at all possible so that I could meet with colleagues face to face, and I filled slots between meetings with admin tasks, which I could do no matter how loud the office was.

When working from home I focused on complex projects or reading research—anything that required quiet concentration time. Using our spare room as a study, I cleared away all distractions until I had a large, clear space in which to work. I started playing relaxing music and decorated the room with flowers to make it a pleasurable place to spend time in.

As at the office, I kept Outlook closed except for my daily email check and did not sign on to our organisation's messenger service. I shared my mobile number with colleagues in case they had an urgent question—but they rarely, if ever, did. I had finally managed to carve out peace and solitude. My happiness soared.

I finally felt that I was truly happy at work and that I had, at last, found balance. No longer feeling at the whim of the agile working policy, I now felt it worked for me. I chose where I was going to work and when. I was available to colleagues when necessary, but no more than that. My time in the office gave me the opportunity to build my social networks and catch up with friends, and because I knew I would soon return to peace and solitude at home, I no longer resented interruptions or distractions from others.

By allocating tasks according to where and when I was working, I also felt that my working routine was in balance with my body. I ticked off difficult and complex tasks during the time when my body was most alert (and tasks were therefore easier) and allowed myself to undertake the less-important tasks when I was less alert. I was on a roll.

REST

y. Leave Work on Time

The last and arguably most important work-related change I made was leaving work on time. More specifically, leaving work on time *every single day*.

Before I got sick, while not working extremely long hours on a regular basis, I was still clocking up to fifty-plus hours a week—and even more if you count the disrupted sleep and constant rumination about work issues while at home. Such hours may or may not be difficult for other people, but for me they were disastrous.

I don't deal well with tiredness, and even working thirty to sixty minutes extra a day disproportionately impacted my health and well-being. And some days I did work later, occasionally to midnight. I began to feel more and more tired and stressed.

Tiredness is a very easy but serious trigger for my mental illness. When I'm tired I lose perspective, become more emotional, and feel less able to cope. I lose the ability to see the big picture, become tangled up in the details, and work longer to try to work myself out of the hole I've dug for myself. And when I do finally arrive home, I bore my husband senseless talking about work. I can't let anything go.

Before I got sick, work had started to become everything to me. It had become an increasingly large part of my identity, and successes (or lack thereof) at work therefore disproportionately affected my sense of self-worth and self-esteem. When deemed to be "average" at my performance review, I felt devastated. I felt "average" as a person.

Taking time off sick gave me the opportunity to regain perspective, but I hold my hands up and admit it took weeks to find. I needed the whole two months to find balance again, and when I eventually found it, I wasn't going to let it go easily.

I realised I had allowed work to take over my life and that health and happiness were more important. Friendships and family were more important than work. For me, work was now just a job, and it had to stay that way.

So I vowed to work my hours and only my hours. If I couldn't do my job in that time, then I would alert my manager to the fact that there was an unmanageable workload and that we would need to deprioritise some activities. But that was easier said than done.

When I initially returned to work, I was working half days so as to not exhaust myself, so leaving work on time was relatively easy because I had my own routine to begin with. But as I slowly increased my hours to full time, the temptation to work later grew.

It was so hard to resist! Every time I packed up to leave at five thirty, the demon on my shoulder told me I was slacking and that I wasn't doing my job well enough. I thought I would be judged by my colleagues. I felt I wasn't doing my job in a determined- or committed-enough way.

But I also knew that in order to remain happy and healthy enough to keep my job, I had to take time in the evening to rest, recharge my batteries, and retain my hard-fought-for perspective. After all, it was a marathon, not a sprint. So I kept my evenings free.

And it felt marvellous. Whole evenings stretched out in front of me to do with as I wished. If I wanted to socialise, I had the time and energy to see friends. I had time to paint and draw. I had quality time with my husband. My overall stress levels remained low, and I was able to see the bigger picture more easily.

Work was easier as I wasn't getting lost in the details. I was able to take a step back and be more objective about decisions. I didn't take work or things that happened at work as personally, and I didn't rely on work for my sense of self-esteem. Instead, my self-esteem came from myself plus the other activities I now had time to do outside of work. I felt balanced.

z. Take Breaks

Just as important as leaving work on time was taking breaks during the day, particularly a lunch break. After all, you really have to pace yourself if you're going to run that marathon. I had rationally known the value of a lunch break before I got sick, but the reality was that I rarely took one, instead eating at my desk. Perspective and energy had deserted me, and I felt my life had turned into an exhausting treadmill of work and sleep.

Taking breaks helped me resist this treadmill effect. I often found solutions to problems that had persistently nagged at me when I stood up and left my desk. I communicated, connected, and collaborated more with colleagues because I saw more of them, more often, away from my desk.

I knew that taking regular breaks was helping me to pace my energy and attention, and I felt less tired and more attentive as a result. I did my work better, faster, and to a higher quality. My memory improved. I made connections I may not have made before.

In short, I was working less but achieving more in a happier and healthier manner. I had finally found my way.

EPILOGUE

One year on, and life has changed dramatically. Work is a positive and productive part of my life, and best of all, it is now contained. I work my hours—and then go home.

With more time to spend at home, I have painted more commissions.[70] My husband and I now train with the Pathways team of Parasnowsport GB[71] and plan to start competing internationally later this year.[72] I have managed to write this book around my full-time day job. I even taught myself how to sew a dress from scratch.

It hasn't always been easy, and I have to practise these steps for positive mental health *every single day*. Just as I visit the gym for my physical health, I paint, journal, and

---

70 www.aliceluetchford.com.

71 The Great British team for disabled skiers and snowboarders who compete in the International Paralympic Committee Alpine Skiing and Snowboarding competitions globally.

72 I am my husband's guide. Skiing in front of him, I verbally guide him down the mountain using a microphone headset. We both love it.

do yoga numerous times a week for my mental health. Even now, I still have good days and bad days.

I am not perfect, but now I don't expect myself to be. I'm doing my best, and forgetting the rest. I am more resilient to change and difficult times, and I know immediately which strategies I need to employ when I start to feel a wobble. It's so much easier preventing a wobble than dealing with the crisis when it happens.

When I returned to work, I wanted something positive to come out of my illness and so decided to talk openly about my mental health. (I also felt that by not talking, I was unintentionally contributing to the stigma around mental health.) So I started to talk. And talk some more. And the response has been amazing.

Every third or fourth person I've told has shared their story with me. Dozens of people have thanked me for my openness and honesty around my illness. I have had colleagues and friends approach me for support and tell me that the ideas I've shared have helped. I have talked about mental health during cross-organisational meetings, ensuring it is firmly on the organisation's agenda. And I ended up writing this book.

Writing this book has been a very therapeutic process for me. But more importantly, I wanted to share the steps that I have found to be so helpful.

Because I hope they help you too.

Resources

Books

Graham Allcott, *How to Be a Productivity Ninja: Worry Less, Achieve More and Love What You Do* (2015)

Gillian Butler and Tony Hope, *Manage Your Mind: The Mental Fitness Guide* (2015)

Susan Cain, *Quiet: The Power of Introverts in a World That Can't Stop Talking* (2012)

Carol Dweck, *Mindset: How You Can Fulfil Your Potential* (2012)

Paul Gilbert, *The Compassionate Mind (Compassion Focused Therapy)* (2010)

Marie Kondo, *Spark Joy: An Illustrated Guide to the Japanese Art of Tidying* (2016)

Greg McKeown, *Essentialism* (2014)

Gretchen Rubin, *The Happiness Project (Revised Edition): Or, Why I Spent a Year Trying to Sing in the Morning, Clean My Closets, Fight Right, Read Aristotle, and Generally Have More Fun* (2016)

Organisations

Action for Happiness: http://www.actionforhappiness.org/

Blurt Foundation: http://blurtitout.org/

Depression Alliance: http://www.depressionalliance.org/

Mind: http://www.mind.org.uk/

National Health Service: http://www.nhs.uk/

Royal College of Psychiatrists: information about and resources for depression—http://www.rcpsych.ac.uk/healthadvice/problemsdisorders/depression.aspx

Quiet Revolution (for introverts): http://www.quietrev.com/

Rethink Mental Illness: https://www.rethink.org/

Samaritans: http://www.samaritans.org/

Sane: http://www.sane.org.uk/

ACKNOWLEDGMENTS

There are a huge number of people who have supported me ever since my first depressive episode, aged nineteen. Friends, family, and professionals, I am extremely grateful to all of you. Without you I would not be alive.

I am particularly thankful to Simon Wessely for taking the time to provide me with kind words of encouragement and signposting me in the right direction for the most robust evidence for this book.

I am thankful to James, Emma, Dani, Rachel, Lucy, and Becks for showing such encouragement in my work and insisting I publish this.

I would also like to thank Rachel for her supportive management and help in returning to—and staying in—work.

And as always, thank you, James, for giving me my reason to live.

AUTHOR BIOGRAPHY

A. Luetchford is a full-time social researcher for a national charity. She holds a bachelor's degree in sociology from the University of Nottingham and a master's degree in social research from Goldsmiths, University of London.

After a ten-year battle with depression, Luetchford has decided to speak out about her experience, to play her part in reducing the stigma associated with mental health issues.

Luetchford lives in London with her blind husband, James. Together they ski with Parasnowsport GB's Pathways team. Luetchford is also a part-time artist. You can find her work by visiting her website at www.aliceluetchford.com.